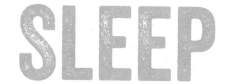

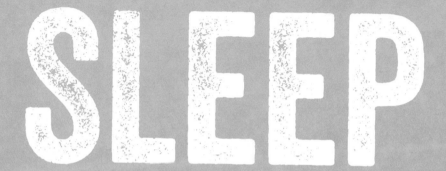

SLEEP

WHAT TO EAT AND DO FOR BETTER SLEEP

ARIANE RESNICK, CNC

The Countryman Press
A division of W. W. Norton & Company
Independent Publishers Since 1923

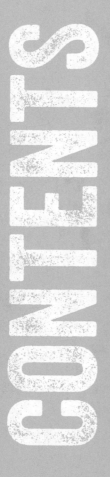

CONTENTS

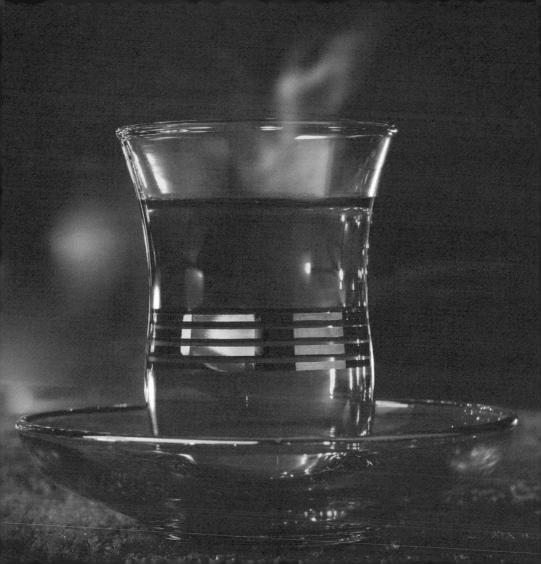

INTRODUCTION

WHY DON'T WE SLEEP WELL ANYMORE, AND WHAT CAN WE DO ABOUT IT?

THE INSOMNIA MONSTER

If you've ever had issues with insomnia, or even if sleeping soundly has never been a challenge for you, you're likely familiar with our cultural lexicon for sleep-inducing foods, from warm milk for its soothing casein and calcium to turkey for its L-tryptophan. In this age of artificial lighting, technological devices we can't seem to pull away from our eyes, and stress levels that often feel outside our control, it's no wonder that about one-third of us suffer from short-term insomnia. As bad as that sounds, what's worse is that nearly 10 percent of the population deals with it long term!

When suffering from insomnia, the temptation is to self-medicate, whether with prescription sleeping pills, over-the-counter sleep aids, or recreational drugs such as alcohol or marijuana. Of course, all of those come with their own risks and side effects, and while they are unlikely to be fatally dangerous, they can be addictive—not to mention that none helps users deal with the causes of insomnia itself.

What Can Help?

Thankfully, there are myriad food-based alternatives that can provide a restful evening and a night that doesn't involve counting sheep, life problems, or anything else! The foods that help people sleep do so for a variety of reasons: they may contain L-tryptophan, an amino acid that regulates serotonin and melatonin; some have casein, the slow-releasing protein in milk that's considered soothing and keeps your muscles sustained throughout the night; others have magnesium, which relaxes the body; still others stimulate glycine, an amino acid that calms the nervous system and improves sleep quality. While the array of nutrients in food that help with sleep is vast, and the range of foods within each category is even broader, my recipes stick to the ones I've just listed, because they offer the most accessible range of foods. It's also easy to understand their science, and I'm looking to help you sleep, but not by boring you into it, after all!

Tryptophan on T-Day Is Real

L-tryptophan, the most well-known sleep nutrient, has been made popular by Thanksgiving turkey and the subsequent "food comas" it induces. Recent research has indicated that we get sleepy after a Thanksgiving feast because of the meal's grandiosity, rather than because of turkey's tryptophan content. Plus, when you couple tryptophan-rich turkey with carbohydrates, which enable our bodies to properly process it, you have a surefire recipe for snoozing. The truth is, many foods are solid competitors to turkey on the tryptophan front: game meats, fish, eggs, and other poul-

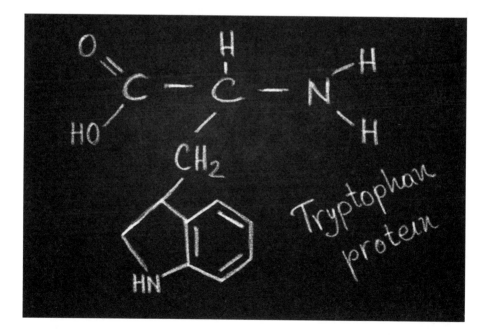

try contain similar amounts, and a single serving of most nuts and seeds have about half the amount. This is good news for the sleep-deprived, because it's easy to make some really delicious late-evening meals with these foods. And just like on Thanksgiving, you'll be better able to absorb the L-tryptophan by eating these dishes with carbs. That's why I offer carby pairing suggestions. Of course, that doesn't mean it's time to bust out the white bread; since any carbohydrate is effective, let's stick to healthful ones such as starchy veggies and whole grains.

Cal/Mag

Calcium and magnesium are sold together as supplements for a good reason: magnesium is needed in order for your body to absorb calcium. While there is much debate over the right ratio of the two in supplement form, when it comes to foods that naturally contain them, no stress is needed. There are no chemical extractions to consider, as nature is doing its thing! Many of the Sleep recipes include dairy and nuts for calcium, and avocados and bananas for magnesium. The two will combine in some recipes, like the No-Machine Ice Cream with just three ingredients (see page 83). Magnesium is often used for anxiety, as its calming effect can chill out even the most tightly wound types.

Glycine, No Lie

Glycine has risen in notoriety as it's come to light that a lot of people are lacking a whole host of essential amino acids, including this one. "Essential" in relation to amino acids refers to those you need to consume because your body doesn't produce them on its own. While our bodies *can* synthesize glycine, often we don't eat the right foods or have a lifestyle that gets our bodies to pump out glycine, and—boom—deficiency. The term for this is a "conditional" amino acid, which means that while we should be able to produce it, we sometimes need to add it to our diet in order to get the amount we need. Glycine, which is super good for getting a solid night's sleep, is readily available in gelatin, bone broth, organ meats, seafood, dairy, and some vegetables and legumes, and I've developed several one-pot meals to cover those bases.

The Case for Casein

If you've ever wondered why a glass of warm milk is the most well-known insomnia cure, your wondering days are over. Milk contains two proteins: whey and casein. Whey is a fast-digesting protein that comprises about 20 percent of milk's overall protein. The remaining 80 percent of milk's protein content is casein, which takes 6 to 8 hours to digest and is the reason, in addition to soothing calcium, that dairy products high in protein, such as milk and

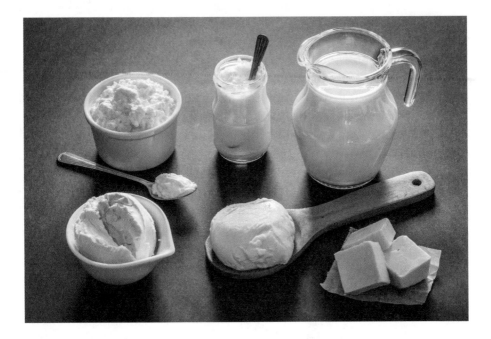

cheese, promote restful sleep. Extracts made from casein are sold in pill form as their own over-the-counter sedative nowadays, because casein is known to help promote relaxation. When it comes to food, the higher the protein content of a dairy product, the more casein it contains. This means that milk, Greek yogurt, and cheese have the most available, which is something to keep in mind if you're on the fence about whether to use a dairy milk or yogurt or a nondairy version in these recipes. (The option is always left up to you!) The most casein-heavy recipe is the queso dip, so for that I definitely recommend not going a vegan cheese route if you want it for its sleep-promoting qualities.

Dairy also contains the feel-good chemicals casomorphins, and the similarity to *morphine* isn't purely coincidental: casein binds to your brain's opiate receptors. If you have ever felt like you are addicted to cheese, this is worth examining. The best relationship with any food is one where you don't feel dependent on it, so it's worth figuring out whether you just love cheese because it's freaking delicious or you have a full-blown habit happening. If you think the latter is the case, remember you can go "cold turkey" for sleep-inducing foods.

THE RECIPES

To make sure you're truly motivated to take this book right into the kitchen with you, I ensured that all the recipes I've provided are lightning fast—or at least moderately quick—to make. They can also be created without chef-level culinary skills or access to elite ingredients. As a certified nutritionist known for my wellness work, it's incredibly important to me that the recipes I recommend contribute to your health, rather than take from it. I believe in focusing on whole foods that can be found at neighborhood grocers, with methods that rely on adding flavor by way of quality ingredients. My motto is that eating and drinking well can, and should, be joyful, and there is no easier way to put that motto to good use than with an ingredient selection that naturally brings joy!

As is my signature style, the recipes in this book are all gluten-free, they can easily be made sugar-free if they aren't already, and they use whole food ingredients. With few exceptions, they're also paleo- and grain-free, and either vegan or have vegan options. I never use starches, gums, or products that contain preservatives. You'll be amazed by how much flavor there is in single ingredients, and by how much delicious relaxation you can add to your evening! Because this side of the book wouldn't make sense focused on single ingredients like *Wake* is, I've divided it into sections of small bites (Nibble), one-pot meals (Spoon), beverages (Sip), and desserts (Sweet). That way, you can choose the right recipe for you based on what you feel like making and when you want to eat or drink it.

Fabulous Fats

In baked goods, unless butter is being used, I typically call for a "neutral" oil. This means a cooking oil that doesn't have any inherent flavor of its own. (An example of a non-neutral oil would be olive oil, which has a strong taste.) There are countless neutral cooking oils on the market, some of which are healthier than others. I recommend avoiding low-quality oils such as generic "vegetable" oil or sunflower oil, as these are high in inflammatory omega-6. Instead, opt for grape seed oil as your cheapest option, or avocado oil if your budget allows for it.

A Note on Sweeteners

Wherever possible, I left the option to you to "sweeten to taste" because desired sweetness is so individual. In testing these recipes, I opted for stevia or Swerve (an erythritol-based sweetener with prebiotics added) wherever possible because I just don't like consuming a lot of actual sugar or recommending that others do so. You can also use monk fruit, a.k.a. lo han, though I don't tend to find it sweet enough. Some natural caloric sweeteners are used, mostly in the forms of honey, maple syrup, or coconut sugar, and when they are liquid, the recipes are based on that quantity of liquid. You are, of course, free to experiment with combos of caloric and non-caloric sweeteners that best serve your own health and taste buds!

THE FINE PRINT

In a world where most of our days are focused on doing and being more, my goal for this side of *Wake/Sleep* is to be a soothing and relaxing deep breath into night. If you have health issues that

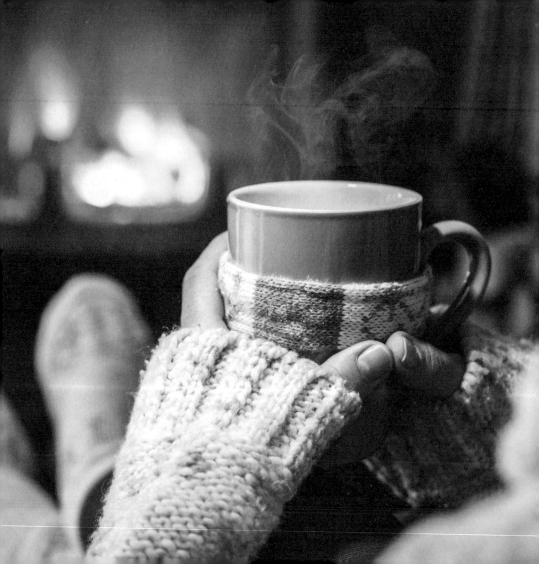

make any ingredients used here questionable for you, check into that thoroughly with your medical professional before using it, and make sure your body is comfortable with small doses of things such as magnesium powder before going big. With a focus on chilling out and settling down by way of healthful, wholesome recipes, I'll help you relax into your evening armed with the tools needed for better slumber. And when you're ready to *Wake*, all you have to do is flip the book over to jumpstart your tomorrow!

DIY Sleep

Having a nighttime ritual is well-known as a smart way to get you in the zzzzone. Because rituals go far beyond food, I've included a selection of DIY ideas that will help you wind down without eating or drinking anything. Similar to the DIY projects in *Wake*, these include essential oils, but relaxing and calming ones instead of energizing ones. The focus is more bath-centric, since that is a common evening activity (see pages 89–90), but there are also other enjoyable self-care tasks, like a face mask (see page 91).

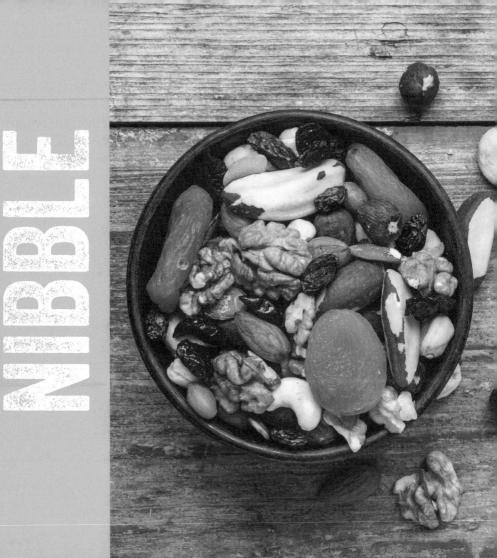

EVENING SNACKING: GOOD OR BAD?

Opinions about whether it's healthy to eat at night are as varied as the options for nighttime snacking itself. It's a topic I myself have vacillated on many times. I go for years never eating after dinner, then I go for years eating a small snack somewhere between 8 and 10 p.m. on the nightly. (Lately I'm an eat-all-the-darned-time-er.) The recipes in this chapter can be eaten any time after breakfast-time, but they are specifically designed to offer healthy options for post-dinner munchies that don't lead to guilt and *do* include ingredients that will help you slumber. That's because evening snacking is real and many people do it, no matter what the professionals say.

The Arguments Against It

The arguments against snacking after dinner are straightforward: you're adding calories to your day. Plain and simple. And if you're into intermittent fasting, you're making your eating window start later the next day. Both of these things are undeniable truths.

If you're the calorie-counting type, you have to factor in late snacks when you eat your earlier meals. I'm not a fan of calorie counting because I don't like the relationship with food that it can create, but I also don't know what life is like in your body, so by all means, handle your food life the way that suits you best!

If you're into intermittent fasting, pay attention to when you're hungriest and plan accordingly. For me, IDGAF if I eat in the morning—coffee, either bulletproof or with about a quarter cup (no joke) of heavy cream, is to me the perfect morning meal. So I'd rather eat my first meal in the afternoon, and thus I feel free to snack later into the evening stress-free, because I know I don't care about morning eating anyway.

My best advice? Choose whether to snack later based on what you eat throughout the day and when you most enjoy eating. If you've joined the no-snacking club, pair a couple of these recipes to create a light evening meal. You'll see in some of the recipes' notes that they contain ingredients that work best in conjunction with other dishes, so that's a pretty functionally fun task.

The Arguments for It

If you go to bed super hungry, it can wake you up at night, which sounds fairly miserable. In fact, feeling stressed about when you eat or don't eat creates cortisol, the stress hormone that can damage your adrenals if it's being produced at inopportune times.

That, in turn, screws with your adrenal system and your sleep. A small snack after dinner prevents this, and if you're eating foods that help relax you, you're doing your adrenal glands a good deed instead of a harmful one.

Additionally, there is the issue of glycogen. This is the form of glucose supplied by your liver that your muscles use to create adenosine triphosphate (ATP), the chemical compounded needed for energy at the cellular level. Eating foods that replenish glycogen, such as honey or starchy vegetables, before bed, can lead to more restful sleep, because your blood sugar won't drop while you are asleep. It can also lead to better brain function. There are a ton of recommendations for having honey before sleep out there in internetland, but I couldn't find a single study on the use of honey before bed for improved sleep, so do note that while replenishing glycogen is a proven good thing, the evidence at this point is purely anecdotal when it comes to honey specifically.

RECIPES

EASY HERB MEATBALLS

Meatballs are generally considered daunting by a lot of cooks because they have so many ingredients, and if you don't get the balance just right, you'll end up with a ball that's either too bready or too soft to work with. People are always shocked when I feed them these yummy meatballs and then they find out they're made with nothing but meat and herbs. These are the meatballs used in the Italian wedding soup that my client P!nk professed to be her favorite dish ever.

All meat contains tryptophan, and in fact pork has even more than poultry, even though turkey is the meat famous for it. Feel free to use a mix of meats so you achieve the flavors you love best. Same goes with herbs: mix them up, use what you have on hand, and get creative! For maximum drowsiness, this dish is best served with a carb-heavy dish, such as Baked Sweet Potato Fries (page 28) or Spiced Roasted Chickpeas (page 27), to help your body activate the L-tryptophan.

MAKES 24 MEATBALLS

INGREDIENTS

- 1 pound (2.2 kg) ground beef, bison, pork, dark turkey meat, or a combo

- ¾ cup (30 g) finely chopped fresh herbs: any combo of parsley, dill, basil, cilantro, rosemary, savory, sage, thyme, tarragon, mint, and/or marjoram

- ¾ teaspoon salt, or more to taste

- ⅛ teaspoon ground black pepper

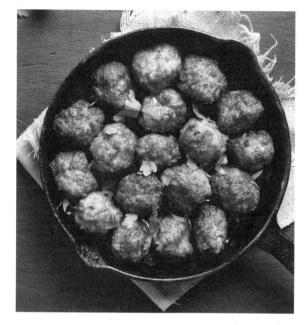

INSTRUCTIONS

1. Preheat the oven to 425°F (220°C).

2. Combine all the ingredients, adding water 1 teaspoon at a time if the mixture is too thick to work with, and form into about 24 miniature meatballs by hand.

3. Roast the meatballs on a cookie sheet 18 to 20 minutes, or until cooked through.

SALMON CREAM CHEESE FLOWERS

Salmon is so special that entire sleep studies have been conducted about it. The results show that this fish does, indeed, help you sleep better. Science says so. Beyond its tryptophan, salmon is a top food source for vitamin D. On the one hand, you need vitamin D for your overall health, and on the other, it improves sleep quality. Note that wild salmon has more vitamin D than farmed, so you'll get more benefits if you go wild. Cream cheese is smoked salmon's natural long-term partner as far as taste pairings go. While it has less casein than firm cheeses, cream cheese still offers calming calcium and circadian-rhythm-regulating vitamin A, both of which will help in your battles against the Insomnia Monster.

MAKES 4 SERVINGS

INGREDIENTS

8 slices smoked salmon   ½ cup (115 g) cream cheese

INSTRUCTIONS

1. On a flat surface, lay out the smoked salmon slices.

2. Press 1 tablespoon of the cream cheese onto each slice, spreading it from one edge to as far across the slices as possible with your fingers or the back of a spoon.

3. Starting at one side, roll up the slice. Use your fingers to pull open the edge that has no cream cheese so it resembles a cut rose. If it does not stand up on its own, slice off the bottom with a knife.

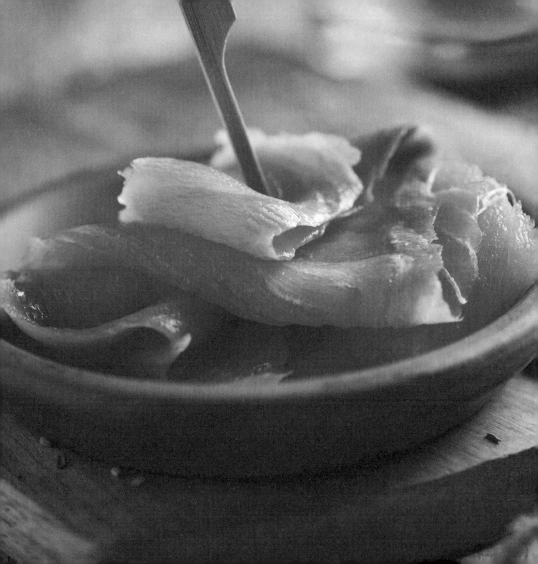

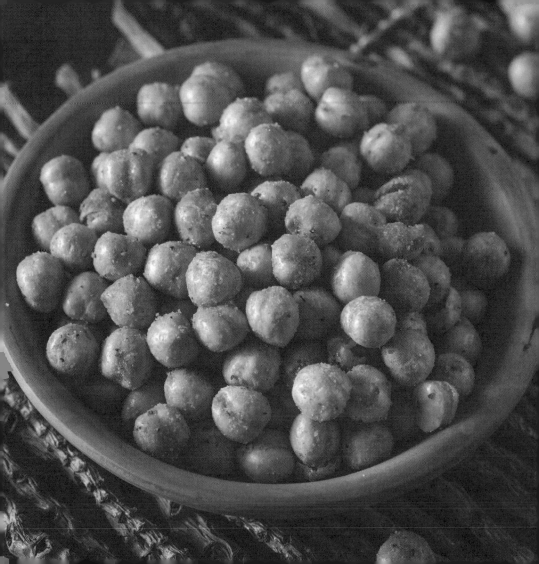

SPICED ROASTED CHICKPEAS

This is an excellent nighttime snack if you find nuts and seeds too heavy for the evening, or if you want something that has a good carb-y feel without having refined carbs. Chickpeas are good for sleep because of their vitamin B6, which helps your body produce serotonin. Since serotonin then converts to melatonin, chickpeas aid in sleep through this two-step process. Feel free to try these with ginger and coconut sugar for a tropical take, or a simple all-purpose seasoning blend. If going for easier digestability, choose digestion-enhancing spices such as fennel, cayenne, or mint.

MAKES 2 CUPS (318 G)

INGREDIENTS

2 cups (318 g) cooked chickpeas

4½ teaspoons neutral oil, such as avocado or grape seed

1 teaspoon chili powder

½ teaspoon salt

¼ teaspoon ground black pepper

INSTRUCTIONS

1. Preheat the oven to 375°F (190°C).

2. Mix all the ingredients together in a mixing bowl, then spread onto a parchment-lined cookie sheet.

3. Roast until golden and chewy, about 20 minutes.

BAKED SWEET POTATO FRIES

Anyone who knows me knows that my eating habits are a little (or a lot!) quirky. I often eat single foods instead of meals, and I have weird spells of eating a two-food combo for ages. A few years ago, I ate these baked fries dipped in mustard a couple times a day . . . for several months. Not only are they easy to make and crazy yummy, sweet potatoes are high in muscle-relaxing potassium. They're also a good source of complex carbohydrates, so they make a perfect pairing with foods that are high in tryptophan, such as the Easy Herb Meatballs (page 22), that need to be eaten along with carbohydrates to activate the tryptophann's sleepy magic.

MAKES 3 TO 4 SERVINGS

INGREDIENTS

1 tablespoon neutral oil, such as avocado or grape seed

3 cups (435 g) sweet potato cut into ¼-inch-wide slices

(about 1 large or 2 small sweet potatoes)

½ teaspoon salt

INSTRUCTIONS

1. Preheat the oven to 415°F (212°C).

2. Drizzle half of the oil onto a parchment-lined cookie sheet, then place the sweet potato slices on the parchment, drizzle with the remaining oil, and sprinkle with the salt.

3. Roast until browned, about 30 minutes, flipping halfway through.

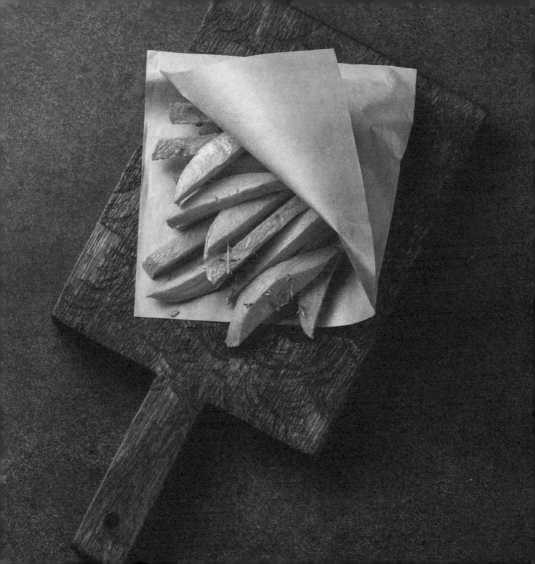

LAVENDER HONEY ALMONDS

The smell of lavender is famous for its soothing, calming effect. When you eat it, you can't help but ingest the aroma, so getting those bennies is straightforward. Lavender also has calcium, which helps you chill out, as well as vitamin A, which regulates circadian rhythm.

Almonds are great not only for their magnesium and tryptophan, but also for controlling ghrelin, a.k.a. the hunger hormone. They can literally help you eat less food overall by improving your sense of satiety.

Honey helps to replenish glycogen, a fuel that your liver stores, which we discussed on page 21. Having enough glycogen right before bed means that your body produces the right amounts of stress hormones throughout the night, which leads to more restful sleep.

MAKES 4 SERVINGS

INGREDIENTS

½ teaspoon coconut oil

½ cup (70 g) raw almonds

½ teaspoon dried lavender flowers

¾ teaspoon honey

Pinch salt

INSTRUCTIONS

1. In a sauté pan over medium heat, melt the coconut oil, then add the almonds.

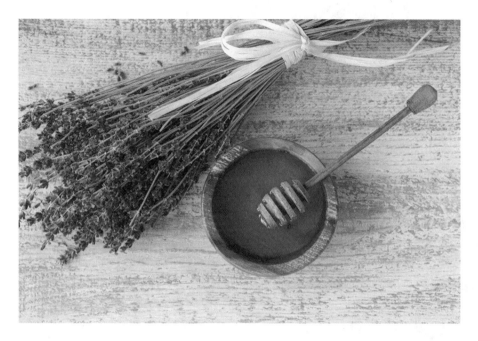

2. Toast the almonds until beginning to darken, then add the lavender, honey, and salt.

3. Sauté for 1 to 2 additional minutes, stirring until evenly coated.

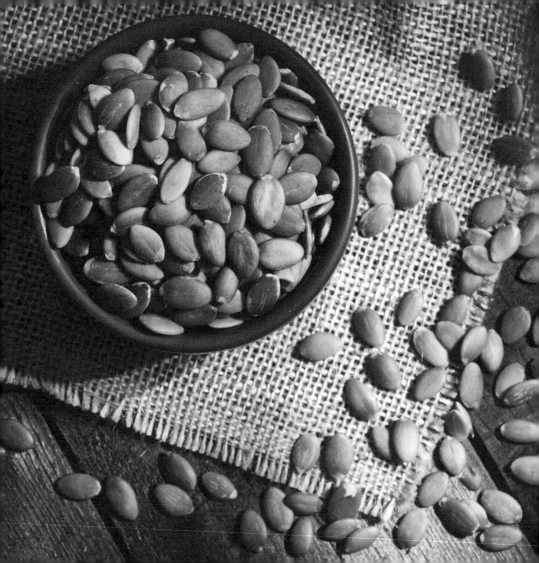

PUMPKIN SPICE PUMPKIN SEEDS

They've been called "the new warm milk," so it should come as no surprise that pumpkin seeds get their own recipe. They have tryptophan, they have the zinc that helps your body convert that tryptophan into serotonin, and they're even good for your sex drive—why not add another evening activity that helps improve sleep!? Pumpkin pie spice includes cinnamon, which helps lower blood sugar, ginger and allspice to aid in digestion by stimulating digestive acids while preventing bloating, and nutmeg, which itself has a directly calming and muscle relaxing effect by way of its sleep-inducing chemical called trimyristin.

MAKES 8 SERVINGS

INGREDIENTS

½ teaspoon coconut oil

1 cup (130 g) pumpkin seeds

1 teaspoon pumpkin pie spice

½ teaspoon sugar or coconut sugar

Small pinch salt

INSTRUCTIONS

1. In a sauté pan over medium heat, melt the coconut oil, then add the pumpkin seeds.

2. Toast for 1 to 2 minutes, until beginning to darken, then add the remaining ingredients.

3. Sauté for an additional 1 to 2 minutes, stirring until evenly coated.

NUTTY SEED CRUMBLE TOPPING

Love the crunch of bread crumbs, but hate that they add calories to a dish without contributing any nutrition? Enter this nutty seed crumble topping, which can be used as a coating for protein or produce before baking. Nuts and seeds in general have good amounts of tryptophan, but pumpkin seeds also contain zinc, which helps the brain convert tryptophan into serotonin. The body then converts that serotonin into melatonin, and boom, you're sleeping better! I've added cashews into the seed mix because I love their richness, as well as their unsaturated fats, which, by the way, improve serotonin levels. Once you've made this topping, it's shelf stable for the life of the seeds/nuts, and any extra can be stored until ready for use.

MAKES 5 TO 6 SERVINGS

INGREDIENTS

¼ cup (35 g) pumpkin seeds

¼ cup (40 g) sesame seeds

¼ cup (40 g) chopped cashews

¾ teaspoon salt

⅛ teaspoon ground black pepper

INSTRUCTIONS

Mix all the ingredients together in a mixing bowl.

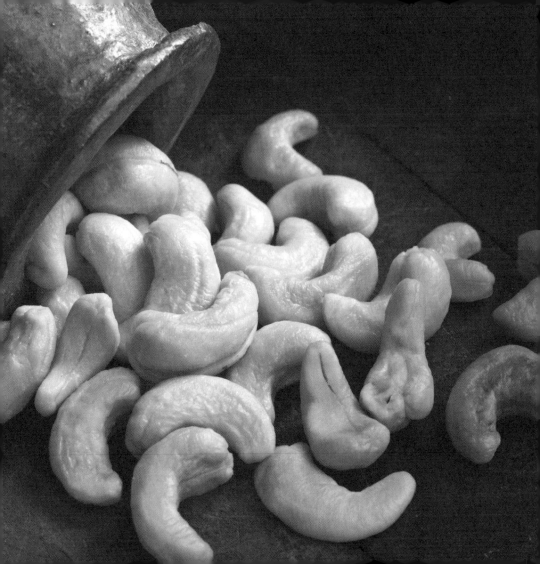

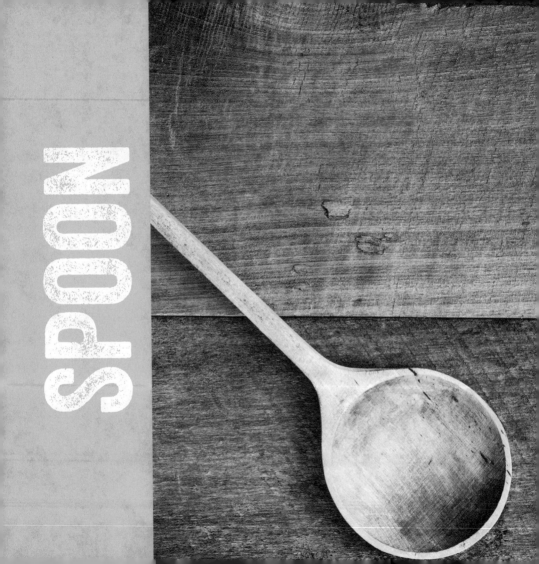

SPOON

DINNER IS UNQUESTIONABLY A THING

Unlike the ever-so-controversial nature of Nibble, with its tough and poignant questions about whether having an evening snack is the right life choice for you, there's no question that we all eat, and need to eat, dinner. Evening meals are the center point of families (or at least they were when I was growing up—I'm a forty-year-old single lady, though, so I can't be trusted on this one) as well as a good reason for get-togethers. (The latter I can be trusted about, and I can confidently tell you that inviting friends over for dinner always, always makes them happy, no matter what is served.)

HOW MANY POTS?

One pot—that's all you need to make any of the Spoon dishes! These recipes were chosen because they are weeknight-friendly, meaning they won't cost a fortune or take your entire night to prepare. The lists of ingredients are noticeably longer than in other chapters, but that's mostly because of all the yummy spices they use. You can trust that these dishes are all quick to put together, take no more than 5 to 10 minutes of chopping, and don't require much maintenance as they cook, either. This means you can start relaxing earlier!

THE COMFORT FACTOR

It's no coincidence that these dishes all err on the dippable, softer side. There is so much to be said for the emotional component of eating, from the textures that comfort us to the smells that remind us of childhood. No matter what your upbringing or cultural background, porridge-like consistencies and broths are the staples of comfort food the world over. While each recipe has ingredients that will assist in sleep, they also have aromas, textures, and flavors designed to help put you in the warm-and-fuzzy zone on every possible level. Those evening relaxation feels are guaranteed to make you happier and calmer before the chemical components in the food even have a chance to work.

LATER, GATOR

While recipes like the coffee drinks in *Wake* make only one portion, these Sleep Spoons make quite a few more. The reason for that is twofold: for one thing, it's kind of hard to make a tiny serving of

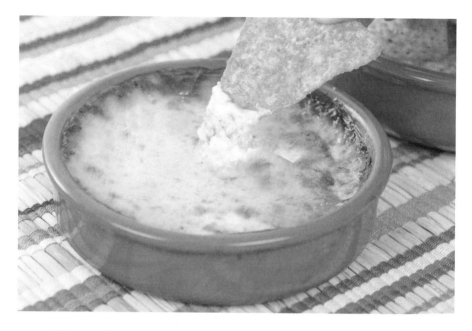

a multifaceted dish. Using a quarter of a jalapeño or a single floret of broccoli leads to a lot of waste, as well as a lot of effort for very little yield. If you have a big group, great—these dishes will be gobbled up all at once. But if it's just you or you plus one, don't worry—they all keep well! Just refrigerate and reheat leftovers when you're ready to enjoy them next. I'm a big fan of making lots of food a couple evenings in a row, then riding high on leftovers swapped back and forth for the next few days.

QUESO DIP

Cheese, glorious cheese! How better to enjoy it than melted in a pot? This fondue-esque recipe even does a better job than fondue at keeping the cheese ooey, gooey, and spreadable as it cools. I'm a huge fondue fan, and queso (as in the dip, and not just Spanish for *cheese*) in particular has a couple bonuses: beyond working better as a party snack that can sit around for a hot (or, well, cooling) minute without congealing, it has some spice to boost your metabolism.

Without question, queso is a high-fat food, and whenever you consume foods high in fat, the best thing you can do for your metabolism is add some heat to them. I chose a pepper jack cheese, partly for its heat and partly because hard cheeses have a high-protein content, meaning plenty of sleep-inducing casein. The fresh chiles and chipotle powder ensure sufficient spice, but you can scale back or swap out any element that's beyond your taste buds. Serve this with your favorite dipping vehicle; it works well with crudités, chips, crackers, and anything else you dream of dipping.

MAKES 6 TO 8 SERVINGS

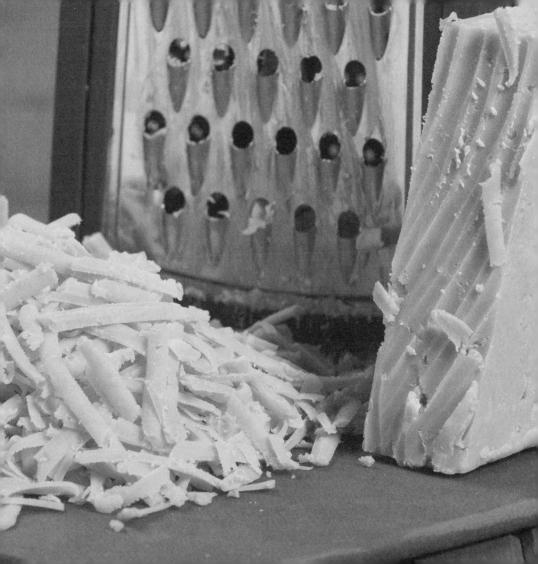

INGREDIENTS

1 tablespoon butter

1 cup (125 g) diced onion

3 tablespoons diced jalapeño

¾ cup (115 g) diced
Anaheim chile

1 tablespoon minced garlic

½ teaspoon paprika

½ teaspoon cumin

1 cup (240 ml) milk

8 ounces (225 g) grated
cheddar

8 ounces (225 g) pepper
jack cheese

1 teaspoon cornstarch mixed
with 1 teaspoon water

1 teaspoon salt, or to taste

Pinch chipotle powder, optional

INSTRUCTIONS

1. In a large saucepot over medium-high heat, melt the butter, then add the onion and chiles and sauté for 10 minutes.

2. Add the garlic, paprika, and cumin, and sauté for 2 additional minutes.

3. Add the milk and cheeses and turn the heat to low. As the cheese begins to melt, stir in the cornstarch-water slurry and stir well.

4. Once fully melted, taste, then add salt and chipotle, if using.

BROCCOLI CORN CHOWDER

Vegetables aren't usually heralded as great for sleep. Much of that comes down to the comfort factor. A warm glass of milk sure makes you think of cozy blankies, while broccoli stalks remind you of getting in trouble at the dinner table for not wanting to eat them. Now that you've grown up a bit, hopefully you enjoy eating vegetables more, or you can at least appreciate that they are full of valuable compounds for sleep. Case in point: corn has melatonin and broccoli has tryptophan. Since tryptophan needs to be eaten with carbs, corn's high content of those is a bonus, as it helps you reap broccoli's sleep powers in addition to providing its own. There's actually more tryptophan available in broccoli once it's been boiled, so this soup is kind of perfect because you're also eating that boiled liquid, and no vitamins are lost like they would be in boiled broccoli.

MAKES 6 TO 8 SERVINGS

INGREDIENTS

4½ teaspoons olive oil

½ cup (65 g) diced onion

4 cups (360 g) broccoli florets

3 cups (435 g) corn kernels (frozen or fresh)

2 tablespoons minced garlic

6 cups (1.4 L) vegetable broth

1 teaspoon Old Bay seasoning

½ teaspoon paprika

1 teaspoon salt

2 tablespoons chopped fresh basil

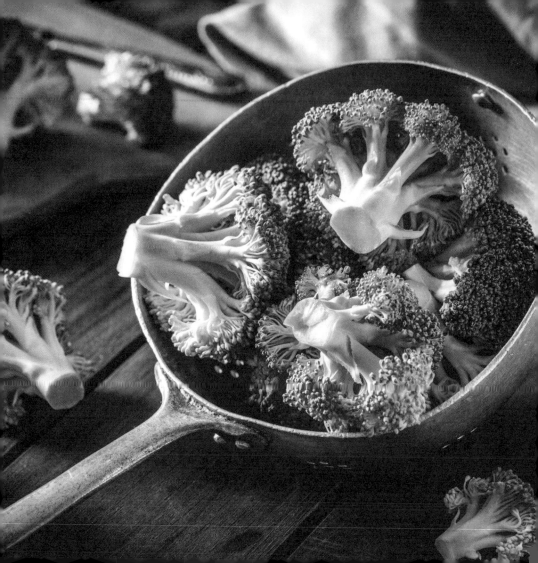

INSTRUCTIONS

1. In a stock pot over medium-high heat, heat the olive oil, then add the onion and sauté until barely golden, about 10 minutes.

2. Add all the remaining ingredients and bring to a boil.

3. Reduce the heat and simmer for 5 to 10 additional minutes, until the broccoli is soft.

TURKEY (OR CHICKEN) STEW

This recipe can also be made with chicken breasts without sacrificing any healthfulness or taste. That said, if bone-in turkey breasts are available, give it a try that way!

For veggies, I encourage you to think outside the potato. There are so many scrumptious root vegetables out there. Parsnips are even sweeter than carrots and just as easy to work with. Celery root, once you cut away the furry outside, rounds out dishes with an amazingly deep and rich vegetal charm. Whatever root veggies you choose, they all have enough carbs to get your body to utilize that lovely, snoozy L-tryptophan in turkey or chicken, so please do experiment.

MAKES 6 TO 8 SERVINGS

INGREDIENTS

1 tablespoon butter or olive oil

1 bone-in turkey breast or 3 bone-in chicken breasts

½ cup (65 g) diced onion

3 cloves garlic, sliced

3 cups (350 g) root vegetables cut into 1-inch (2.5 cm) cubes

3 cups (720 ml) bone broth, vegetable broth, or water

¼ cup (60 ml) balsamic vinegar

2 tablespoons tomato paste

2 bay leaves

1 tablespoon dried or 2 sprigs fresh thyme

1 teaspoon dried or 2 leaves fresh sage

1 teaspoon salt, or to taste

¼ teaspoon ground black pepper

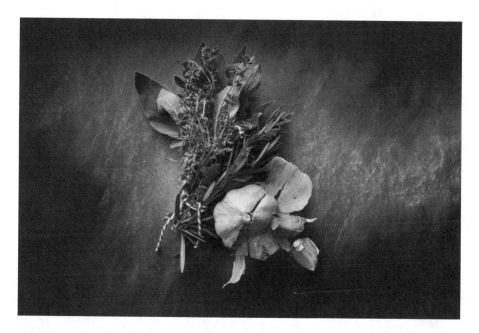

INSTRUCTIONS

1. In a soup pot over medium-high heat, heat the butter, then add the turkey or chicken breast(s) and sauté until the skin is golden, about 5 minutes, turning once.

2. Add the onion and garlic and sauté for 2 additional minutes.

3. Add all the remaining ingredients and bring to a boil.

4. Reduce to a simmer and cook until the poultry falls off the bone, about 1 hour.

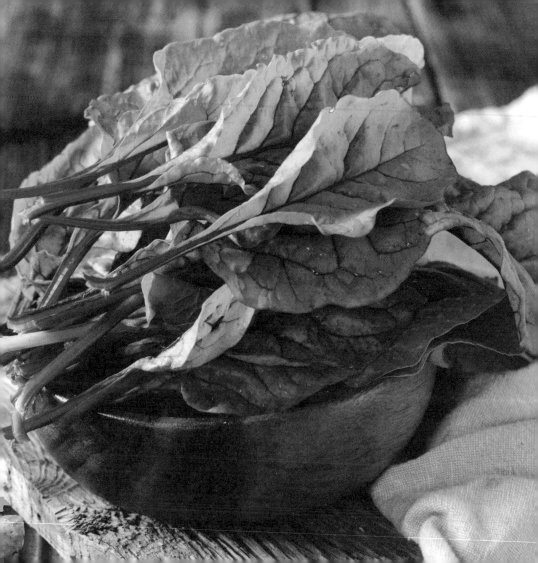

RICE & GREENS SOUP

I think it is important to have a few recipes up your sleeve that taste like you spent a lot of time in the kitchen, when really, you spent about 10 minutes total there. This soup makes excellent use of leftover rice, and baby greens take but a moment to cook. Leafy greens such as spinach and chard lend the sleep-promoting effects of potassium, magnesium, and calcium. The carbohydrate content of the rice makes it a perfect pair to any tryptophan-containing recipe, as it will help your body absorb that sleepy amino acid. Bone broth makes it hearty, with gut-healing benefits, while vegetable stock will yield a lighter result; choose what works best for you.

MAKES 6 TO 8 SERVINGS

INGREDIENTS

6 cups (1.4 L) bone broth or vegetable stock

4 cups (80 g) mixed baby greens such as spinach or chard

1 cup (200 g) cooked rice

1 tablespoon Italian seasoning

1 teaspoon salt

INSTRUCTIONS

In a soup pot over medium-high heat, bring the broth to a boil. Add all the remaining ingredients, reduce the heat, and simmer until the greens are thoroughly wilted, about 2 to 3 minutes.

KITCHARI

This Ayurvedic staple is a basic dish that promotes healing. The spice combo is a complex one, and I just didn't feel right telling you to go buy a dozen different spices that you'd then have to sauté and grind just to make one recipe. Enter curry powder, which, no matter what brand you buy, has at least most, if not all, of the spices used in kitchari. I also used cinnamon, because most people have it on hand and the flavor rounds out the dish. The combo of rice and mung beans is a perfect one, since the rice will enable your body to use the tryptophan in the beans—no need to combine this recipe with any other for best results! Bonus: Kombu, also known as kelp, is a seaweed that's great for your thyroid. It also adds an umami quality that gives this dish a well-rounded flavor.

MAKES 4 TO 6 SERVINGS

INGREDIENTS

2 tablespoons ghee, butter, or coconut oil

2 tablespoons curry powder

1 teaspoon cinnamon

1-inch (2.5-cm) piece kombu, optional

1 cup (195 g) yellow dal mung beans

1 cup (180 g) basmati rice

1½ teaspoons salt

INSTRUCTIONS

1. In a stock pot over low heat, melt the ghee, then add the curry powder and cinnamon and sauté for 1 minute.

2. Add 6 cups (1.4 L) water and the kombu, if using, and bring to a boil.

3. Rinse the dal and rice until the water runs clear, then add to the pot with the salt.

4. Reduce the heat to a simmer and cook about 45 minutes, until a porridge consistency is reached.

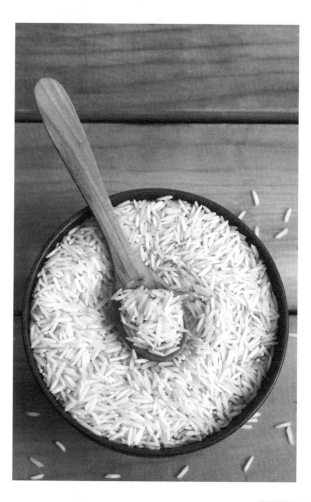

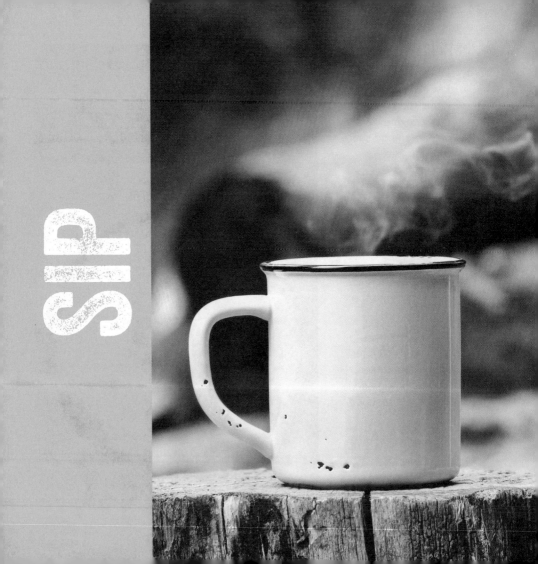

THE MOCKTAIL CROWD

Evening drinks that aren't alcoholic are an under-served category of beverages, with decaf coffee or sparkling water with citrus being the only really popular options in most social settings. As much as I love wine and cocktails, I also understand that not every night is the right night for imbibing. For years now, I've been on a mission to make sure there is no shortage in the world of drinks that don't contain alcohol but do contain healthful, indulgent-seeming ingredients. These are adult drinks that can fit in at a gathering and maybe even make the guy with the Bud Lite a little jealous.

RUNNING HOT & COLD

A glass of warm milk is the quintessential nighttime bevvie; there is something inherently soothing and calming about warm liquids. Because of this, I've included a selection of hot drinks in this chapter. That said, because liquids take longer to move through your digestive system when they're hot, and because summer exists, I also wanted to make sure there are cold drinks to be had. Magnesium powder is an ideal choice for a chilled beverage because it comes in assorted fruity flavors, so I paired it with liquids best served cold, such as sparkling water and tart cherry juice.

WHAT ABOUT DECAF?

Espresso and coffee drinks are an after-dinner offering at nearly every restaurant, and some people even just order regular because they can handle having caffeine late into the night and still fall asleep without an issue. I'm not one of those people, as I would be tapping my toes and cursing the world from my bed at 4 a.m. I've tried decaf drinks, but in my experience, that small amount of caffeine (because "decaf" does not mean "no caf") is still too much for me, and it heavily impacted my sleep quality. The average 8-ounce (240 ml) serving of decaf coffee (which is a standard good-size mug's worth) has 12 or 13 milligrams of caffeine. That's not a ton, but it is like having a hardy serving of chocolate, and if you're also getting the Death by Chocolate dessert, you will indeed be well and truly caffeinated. If that's not a problem for you, feel free to try some of the drinks on the *Wake* side but use decaf at night! As for me, I'll stick with this chapter's choices.

THE LOWDOWN ON COFFEE SUBS

Coffee substitutes are usually made from roasted grains, which are then powdered. They are created from an assortment of plant items, such as chicory, dandelion, rye, and barley. There's also a fairly new coffee sub available that's made out of maya nuts, a.k.a. capomo, which can be brewed either in a French press like cof-

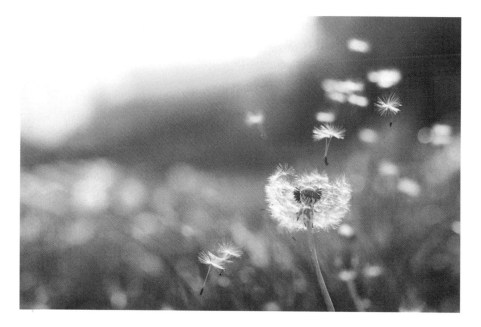

fee or steeped like tea. Despite often being made from glutinous grains, roasted-grain coffee substitutes will usually be labeled gluten free. If you have concerns about that, pick one that is not made with the gluten culprits wheat, barley, or rye. Even with that limitation, there are lots to choose from.

As good as coffee subs are, there's only one recipe in this chapter that utilizes one, which was a conscious choice on my part. I didn't want to give you a bunch, because you can make any of the coffee recipes on the *Wake* side with a sub instead. I felt like a mocha free of both chocolate and coffee was the most important sleepy-drink idea I could give you, so I went with that and just that (see opposite page).

RECIPES

NO-COFFEE, NO-CHOCOLATE MOCHA

Back in the 1980s, when we all mistakenly thought fat was bad, the health food world also found fault in chocolate, mostly for being potentially over-stimulating. Enter carob, a noncaffeinated bean that can be ground into a rich powder to use in sweets. It's for sure not chocolate, but it's not half bad, either. It's high in fiber, reduces ghrelin (the hunger hormone), and contains potent antioxidants, all of which really up the health factor of this drink.

My favorite coffee substitute, a.k.a. roasted grain beverage, is Dandy Blend, but any will work—just go heavy with your spoonful(s). Generally, I find the key to a great cup of coffee sub is to use much more than the package instructs so you get a heavier, coff-ier result. Otherwise, I find them all as weak as tea. That's why this recipe calls for two servings to make one serving.

MAKES 1 SERVING

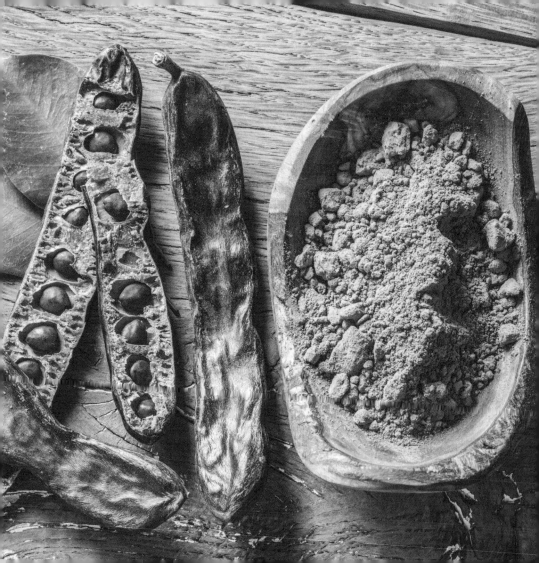

INGREDIENTS

1 tablespoon carob powder

2 servings coffee substitute

1–2 tablespoons heavy cream or coconut creamer

1 cup (240 ml) hot water

INSTRUCTIONS

In a sauce pot over low heat, combine all the ingredients, whisking to ensure the carob powder is smoothly incorporated.

CAL-MAG CHERRY JUICE

It's a given that magnesium powder will help you fall asleep, but both my sous chef and I were legitimately, and literally, floored by how hard and fast we passed out when combining it with tart cherry juice. This is a power-punch of sleepiness, so be sure to drink it at home with your evening hygiene tasks already accomplished. We barely managed to brush our teeth before falling into bed after drinking this!

What makes this such a potent sleeping potion? For one, tart cherries contain high doses of melatonin and have been shown to improve sleep duration, as well as sleep efficiency, meaning you might wake up less throughout the night than normal. Additionally, tart cherry juice is a proven anti-inflammatory that reduces muscle pain in athletes. Since magnesium acts similarly in that respect, this drink is basically a godsend on multiple levels. If you find yourself using the bathroom more quickly in the morning, don't be surprised—helping move things along is another one of magnesium's charms.

MAKES 1 SERVING

INGREDIENTS

1 serving calcium
magnesium powder

1 cup (240 ml) tart cherry juice

INSTRUCTIONS

Dissolve the magnesium powder in small amount of the cherry juice, then add the remaining juice and stir.

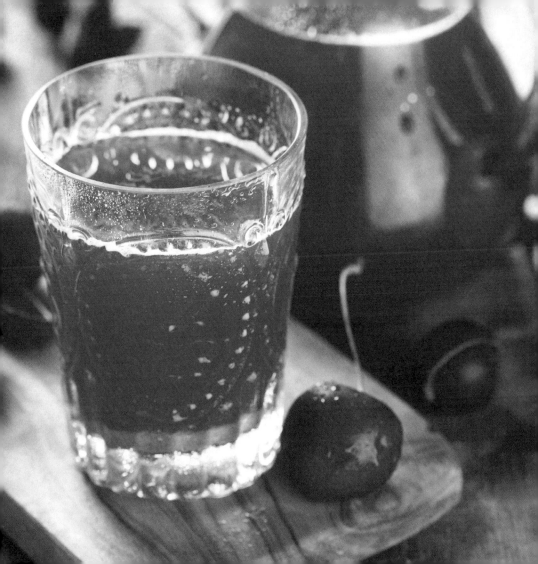

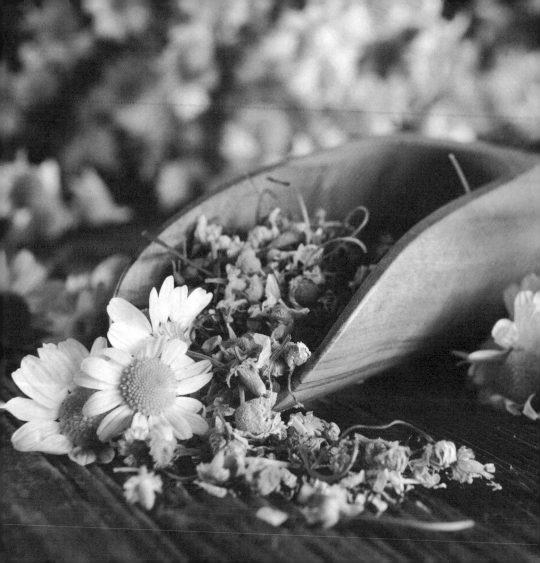

LAVENDER CHAMOMILE SWEET SIPPER

Much like the cherry-magnesium mash-up (see page 60) being wonderfully greater than the sum of its parts, pairing chamomile with lavender makes for a floral explosion of relaxation. But because both are more mild in their sedative abilities than Cal-Mag Cherry Juice, this drink is safe for earlier in the day if you're just looking to chill out. Chamomile provides a statistical reduction in anxiety when tested, and lavender goes even beyond that: silexan, a capsulized preparation of lavender oil, was as effective for calming as benzodiazepines in a six-week double-blind study of both. Honey's ability to soothe and relax tops off this drink that, if you like, can also be consumed hot.

MAKES 1 SERVING

INGREDIENTS

- 1 bag chamomile tea
- 1 teaspoon dried lavender flowers
- ¼ cup (60 ml) nearly boiling water
- 1 teaspoon honey or maple syrup
- ¾ cup (180 ml) cold water

INSTRUCTIONS

1. Steep the tea and flowers in the nearly boiling water for 5 minutes, then add the honey and strain.

2. Add cold water, and ice if desired.

18-KARAT MILK

If there's one drink that's the golden child of the wellness world, it's golden milk. Turmeric lattes are nothing new, having been a staple of Eastern cultures for many a millennium. A potent, earthy, and somewhat sharp-tasting root from the ginger family, turmeric has historically been used as an anti-inflammatory (in addition to being used as a natural coloring). Today we know that's in part thanks to its active anti-inflammatory element curcumin, which can now be purchased as its own extract. Because studies on curcumin in turmeric haven't panned out as well as researchers thought they would, it is speculated that there are likely other active compounds in turmeric that contribute to its effectiveness. No matter what the science is, you can drink this tasty bevvie to reduce pain, increase relaxation, lower blood sugar, and improve digestion. It's also safe to imbibe early in the day, as it won't knock you out. I prefer fresh turmeric root, but I made this with the powder because it's more readily available.

MAKES 1 SERVING

INGREDIENTS

1 cup (240 ml) milk (dairy or non)

½–1 teaspoon turmeric powder (as much as you can tolerate)

¼ teaspoon cinnamon

Sweetener, to taste

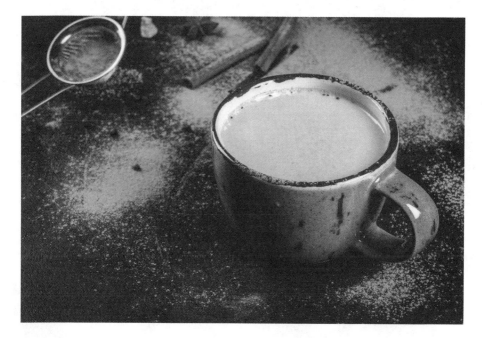

INSTRUCTIONS

1. In a small pot over medium-low heat, combine all the ingredients.

2. Stir to incorporate the cinnamon thoroughly and heat until very lightly steaming.

3. In a small sauce pot over low heat, whisk all the ingredients together well to incorporate the turmeric and cinnamon.

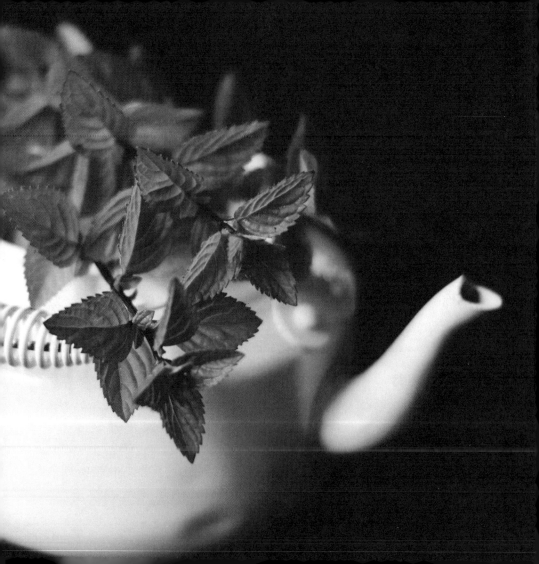

PEPPERMINT TEA LATTE

Stomach-settling peppermint is the perfect after-dinner drink. It reduces gas, assists with digestion (including digestive ailments such as IBS), and relieves stress. It can be invigorating regardless of its relaxing properties, so for this drink I've included valerian, which is used purely to incite restfulness. Valerian has been used since ancient Greek and Roman times as a sedative and relaxant, but interestingly, studies on its effectiveness have been rather inconclusive overall. Some particular studies found that it can lessen the time needed to fall asleep and help with staying asleep, but even in studies where valerian didn't offer much more benefit than a placebo, it also didn't have any major side effects. So while this might not make you pass right out every time, it will settle your stomach and relax you a bit, and there's surely nothing wrong with that!

MAKES 1 SERVING

INGREDIENTS

- 1 bag peppermint tea
- 1 bag valerian tea
- ¾ cup (180 ml) nearly boiling water
- ¼ cup (60 ml) milk (dairy or non)
- Sweetener to taste

INSTRUCTIONS

1. Brew the teas in the nearly boiling water for 5 minutes.

2. Remove the tea bags, add the milk, and sweeten to taste.

CAL-MAG CITRUS SODA

For those who love bubbly carbonated drinks but don't want to drink soda or champagne before bed, this sleepy soda is a choice that's both healthful *and* good at helping get you to bed. Because magnesium and calcium work symbiotically, you can get more benefit from relaxing magnesium powders when they are enhanced with calcium. Plus, the calcium alone is relaxing, as well as great for your bones. Detoxifying lemon or lime juice is a good way to alkalize your body, a.k.a. make it less hospitable to the free radical that can cause illness, and the minerals in sparkling water make it a sounder choice than seltzer, which contains a negligible amount, if any. For a more indulgent soda-pop feel, choose a flavored cal-mag powder such as raspberry or lemon. If you find yourself using the bathroom more quickly in the morning, don't be surprised—helping move things along is another one of magnesium's charms.

MAKES 1 SERVING

INGREDIENTS

1 serving calcium-
   magnesium powder

1 cup (240 ml) sparkling water

2 tablespoons lemon or
   lime juice

Sweetener, to taste

INSTRUCTIONS

Mix the cal-mag powder with a small amount of sparkling water until dissolved, then add the remaining water, citrus juice, and sweetener, if using.

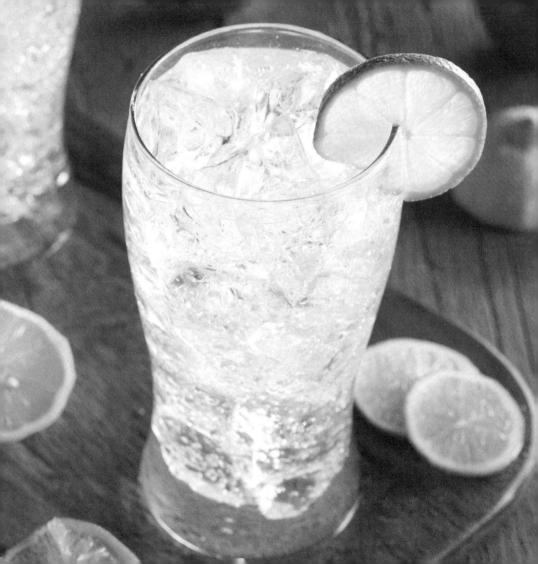

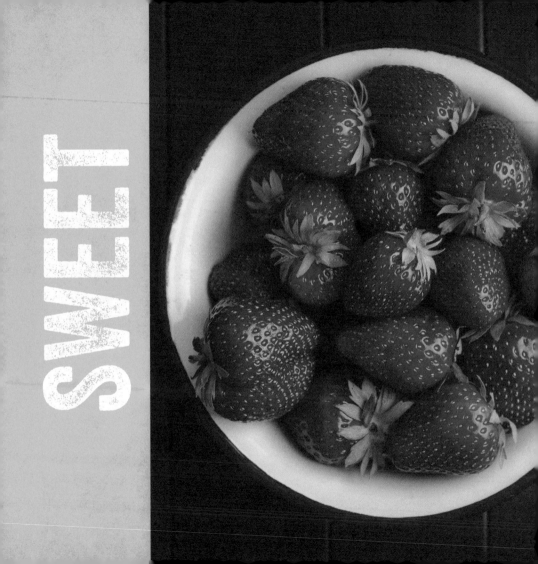

SWEET

THE TIMING

Dessert. It usually happens at night, so wouldn't it be cool if it also led to more restful sleep? While none of these sweet treats will bowl you right on over into dreamland, they all contain ingredients that will make nodding off easier. From a no-machine ice cream that's far lower in added sweetener than a condensed-milk version, to a doughnut rich in fiber and tryptophan, these recipes are sounder choices for an evening sweeter than most packaged products could dream of being.

FIBER FACTORS

Almond flour, coconut flour, and avocado are all fiber-rich ingredients, and I made sure to include fiberlicious elements in the *Sleep* recipes, because studies have shown that people who eat high-fiber diets are able to stay in a state of deep, dreamless sleep (known as "slow-wave sleep") for longer than people who are fiber-poor. Getting enough fiber in a day can also help you to fall asleep 10 to 15 minutes more quickly than you would on a day with insufficient fiber intake. I could go on and on, as there are countless reasons to include enough fiber in your diet, like the fact that it helps your positive gut bacteria thrive, but better sleep is all we need to think about for now.

FRUIT FORWARD

You may notice that the focus here eschews dessert standards such as chocolate—which I found to be a better fit for the *Wake*

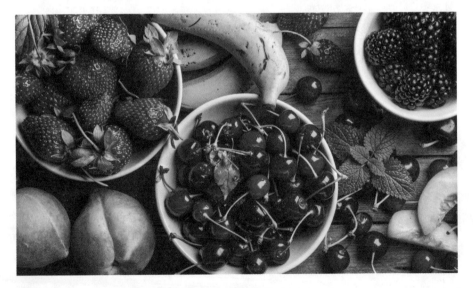

section, due to its caffeine and stimulating effects—and instead uses fruits such as mangoes, avocados, and bananas. That's because, in addition to not having any stimulant effects, these all have a good amount of fiber to offset their natural sugar content. Fiber slows down your body's absorption of sugar, which makes you less likely to get an energetic sugar high at exactly the wrong time of day. And since fruit is sweet to begin with, recipes that use it require less additional processed sweeteners than other desserts with bitter ingredients, such as cocoa that only become sweet when you add sugars and sweeteners.

THE ROLE OF SUGAR

Wherever possible, I chose honey as the sweetener in the *Sleep* desserts because of its positive effect on your body's glycogen stores (see page 21 for more on that). Where a dry sweetener is needed, nighttime is an ideal time to try out a noncaloric sweetener, because unlike cane sugar, it won't spike and then crash your blood sugar. And why is that important? Sugar's up-and-down effect can end up making you hungry again before bedtime. Also, the less sugar you eat, the deeper you are likely to sleep; studies have shown that consuming lots of sugar can lead to lighter, less restful sleep. So keep all that in mind when a recipe gives you the option of using Swerve—a noncaloric, erythritol sugar replacement—instead of sugar.

RECIPES

BANANA PUDDING

I wanted to make a banana pudding that was as simple as could be, but I didn't want it to read as baby food. Mission accomplished with the additions of Greek yogurt and coconut water. Coconut water provides the extra sweetness the bananas needed, and Greek yogurt offers a dollop of protein and calcium with a tiny bit of grown-up tanginess. The bananas themselves contain a solid mix of sleep-inducing compounds: potassium, magnesium, and L-tryptophan. Because they're heavy in carbs, their tryptophan content is available as is, without having to add in more carby foods to activate them. Frozen bananas will work here for more of a "nice cream" (the term used for blending bananas into an ice cream–like treat) vibe, but you might need a food processor instead of a blender, since they are so much more firm than fresh ones.

MAKES 2 SERVINGS

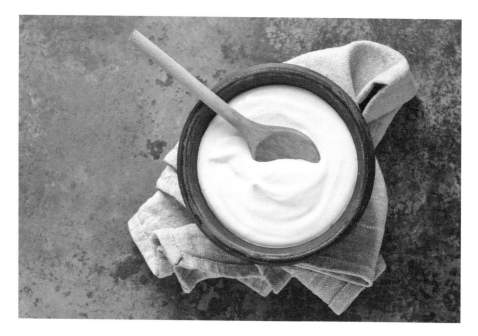

INGREDIENTS

2 small bananas

2 tablespoons coconut water

1 tablespoon Greek yogurt

Small pinch salt

INSTRUCTIONS

In a blender, combine all the ingredients until smooth and creamy.

BAKED PUMPKIN DOUGHNUTS

Similar to bananas, pumpkins contain L-tryptophan and enough carbo-hydrates for said tryptophan to be effective. Almond flour is made purely of almonds, so it offers the same hunger-reducing effects of its whole-nut counterpart, which is always helpful for a late-night snack. Cider vinegar is necessary for fluffiness, but feel free to use white vinegar if you don't have its apple sister on hand. Coconut flour is high in fiber and protein to keep you full, too, and avocado oil is an unsaturated fat that helps your body produce serotonin. Also, hello, what's more exciting than doughnuts late at night?! My life changed when I got a doughnut pan, and I imagine yours will, too.

MAKES 10 DOUGHNUTS

INGREDIENTS

1 cup (240 ml) pumpkin or kabocha puree

1 cup (115 g) almond flour

¾ cup (150 g) sugar, coconut sugar, Swerve, or a combo

⅓ cup (75 ml) neutral oil, such as avocado or grape seed

¼ cup (30 g) coconut flour

¼ cup (60 ml) milk (dairy or non)

2 large eggs

1½ teaspoons pumpkin pie spice

1 teaspoon baking soda

½ teaspoon salt

2 tablespoons apple cider vinegar

INSTRUCTIONS

1. Preheat the oven to 325°F (160°C).

2. In a mixing bowl, combine all the ingredients except the cider vinegar, ensuring no lumps of flour remain.

3. Add the cider vinegar and stir to incorporate thoroughly.

4. Divide the batter into 10 greased doughnut molds.

5. Bake about 20 minutes, until cooked through.

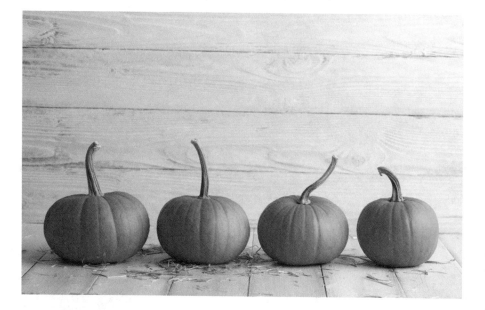

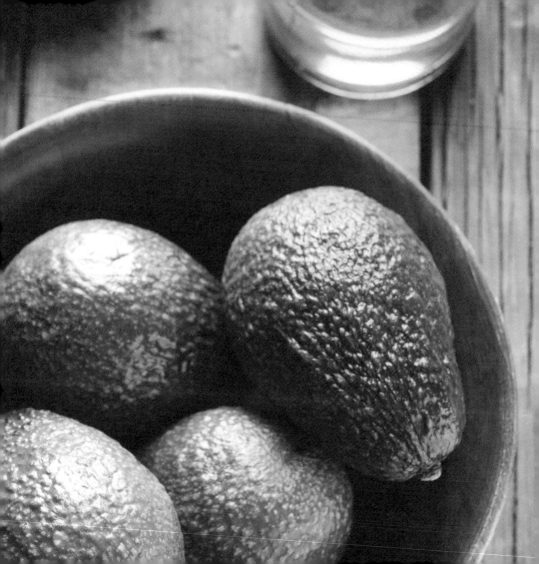

LEMON-LIME AVO MOUSSE

Avocados as dessert is one of my very favorite things in life. That has nothing to do with the fact that the avocado's high unsaturated fat content helps your body produce serotonin, which is then converted to melatonin, but that sure is an added bonus! The real reason I love avos for dessert is that they bring heavy richness to the table while also bringing along enough fiber to help slow the absorption of any caloric sweeteners you add to them. I don't usually recommend cassava products because they are so high in unhealthy starch, but I find cassava syrup a healthier vegan option than agave because it has no fructose. (Fructose isn't a type of sugar you'd want before bed, if at all, due to how quickly it gets stored as fat.) If you're feeling wild on the fruit factor, you can throw in a handful of raspberries or blackberries for a berry-citrus delight.

MAKES 2 TO 3 SERVINGS

INGREDIENTS

- 2 medium avocados, peeled and pitted
- 2 tablespoons lemon juice
- 1 tablespoon lime juice
- ¼ cup (60 ml) honey or cassava syrup
- 2 tablespoons coconut oil

INSTRUCTIONS

In a blender, combine all the ingredients, adding water if needed, until smooth and creamy.

CREAMSICLE SHAKE

On occasion, I surprise myself with an idea that I think can't possibly taste as good as "the real thing," but then totally does. This was one of those ideas! No ice cream is even needed to get that nostalgic two-tone taste, and what's better than an ice creamy dessert that keeps you free of unhealthy indulgence-based guilt? Greek yogurt provides sleepy calcium and casein (as well as tons of protein), and the protein powder slows the blood-sugar spike that comes with fruit and fruit juice. Mangoes have a compound called linalool that reduces stress, so in addition to being good for eyesight, thanks to their lutein and zeaxanthin, they also help you mellow out.

MAKES 2 SERVINGS

INGREDIENTS

¾ cup (190 g) frozen mango

1 cup (240 ml) orange juice

½ cup (120 ml) Greek yogurt

1 scoop vanilla protein powder (I use bone broth protein)

1 teaspoon vanilla extract

INSTRUCTIONS

In a blender, combine all the ingredients until creamy.

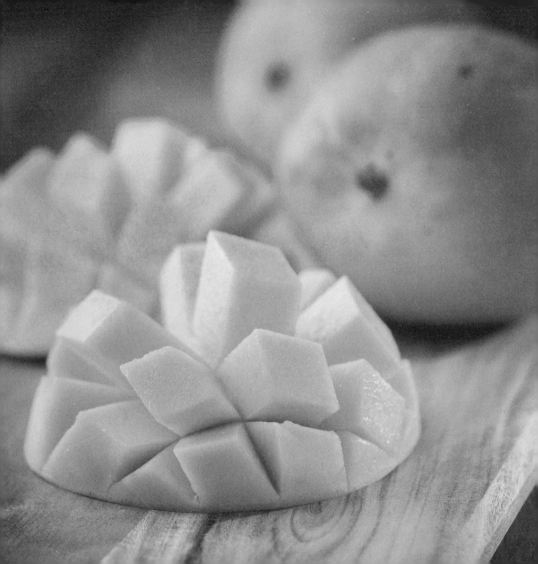

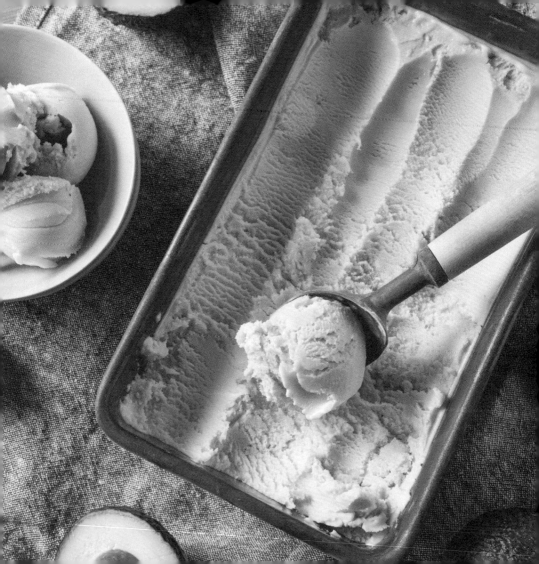

NO-MACHINE ICE CREAM

There is many a recipe out there in internetland for no-machine ice cream, and nearly all of them want you to buy canned condensed milk. Conversely, I do not want you to buy canned condensed milk . . . or at least, I don't want to be the reason you do, because that much sugar before bed is definitely not gonna help you sleep. Avocado, honey, and cream stand a much better chance of taking you to slumbertown. Simply blend up this mixture, throw it in the freezer for a couple of hours, and you have a super delectable treat that's much healthier than canned sugar-milk or most things found readymade in a carton.

MAKES 6 SERVINGS

INGREDIENTS

1 cup (240 ml) heavy cream

1 avocado, peeled and pitted

¼ cup (60 ml) honey

½ teaspoon vanilla extract

Small pinch salt

INSTRUCTIONS

1. In a blender, combine all the ingredients until thick and creamy.

2. Transfer to a freezer-safe container and freeze 2 to 4 hours, or until firm.

DIY

WHAT'S THE BIG DIY-EAL?

If you're at all crafty or have even just visited sites like Pinterest that highlight homemade goods, you definitely know that there are countless recipes for homemade bath and beauty products. While commercial brands will charge by the ounce, or even by the fraction of the ounce, you can often make your own by the pound for far less than an ounce of a single-purchase product. Sure, there are some commercial products worth buying, but the products in this chapter are all so easy to make that you might as well try them out as quick replacements for things you would otherwise have to purchase.

SELF-CARE IS THE NEW BUSY

I'm sure you've heard the term "self-care" thrown around lately. Years ago, as a culture, we got obsessed with being as busy

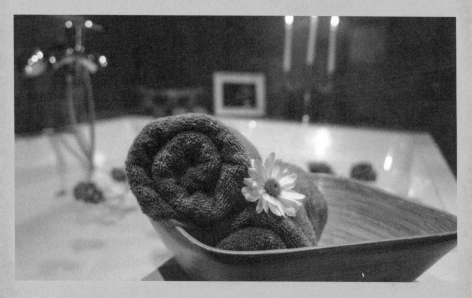

as humanly possible . . . and then, collectively, we got really freaking tired. We tried to backtrack a bit, but most of us found ourselves overscheduled with no way to reduce the loads we'd taken on. Enter self-care, where we schedule in time to, you know, care about ourselves rather than everybody and everything else. Health and beauty are inextricably tied together, so some of the most popular self-care practices that have come into the mainstream are basic beauty routines that could easily go by the wayside in all our busy-ness. But don't think about them in terms of their awesome beauty bennies; think about the calm, soothing opportunities they give you to show yourself a little love.

ROUTINES FOR SLUMBER

Having an evening routine, or ritual, can be a relaxing affair no matter what it is. Studies have shown that starting from infancy, having a set nightly routine leads to waking up less throughout the night. That, in turn, leads to being well rested and therefore more functional tomorrow. Even the small act of setting a nightly bedtime and sticking to it can improve your sleeping life! Something that actually has sleep-inducing effects, such as a bath, is an excellent way to both get into a healthy habit and improve your sleep quality.

JUST BREATHE

Scents have extremely evocative powers. They can be agents of nostalgia, calling up memories that go all the way back to childhood. The neurological responses we have to different smells are definitely intense, and it has been shown that a smell will trigger stronger emotions and more vivid recollections of an event than an image will. Our sense of smell is more acute and more sensitive than any of our other senses, so it isn't too big of a surprise that certain scents can calm our minds and sooth us into restfulness.

OIL FOR EASE

There are plenty of ways to get a scent into your DIY bath and beauty products, but the purest and simplest one is to use essential oils. Essential oils are concentrated versions of plants that have been boiled down . . . and down . . . and down until just a drop or two is enough to have a potent impact. Some oils have a wake-up effect, which you'll learn about in the *Wake* section, while others incite a relaxed response in our bodies and brains. Those are the ones you'll find in this *Sleep* section.

When it comes to picking oils, I prefer non-GMO oils, because you're putting them on your body, and it's always best to breathe in or slather on something full of concentrated pesticides. There are many reputable brands of essential oils, but for some reason, the best ones are multi-level-marketing based and have to be ordered through a human rather than a website or store. My advice here is to generally avoid inexpensive internet-based brands, or generic ones you find at bath and body care shops. In my experience, they just don't smell as good and tend to be cut with other oils. Do your research. It'll be worth it!

YOGURT BATH SOAK

I admit it. I read about yogurt bath soaks, thought they sounded really inventive and interesting, then completely freaked out at the concept when it came time to try it IRL. Thank heavens I found a willing test subject, who let me know after that it was a wonderful experience, and I later became a fan myself. Epsom salts are relaxing because they are made out of magnesium, and yogurt is a good mixer because your skin is porous, so you (honestly, gotta say "presumably" here because there are zero studies on this one) absorb its calcium and casein that way. If

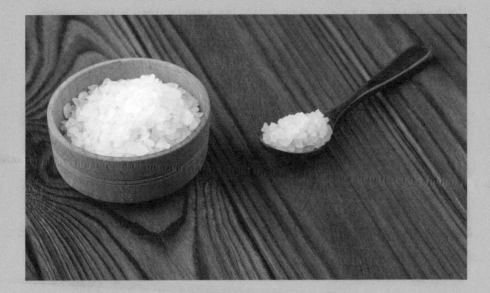

you're female-bodied, this is also a sound way to ensure your internal yeast production stays in check. Feel free to add in any relaxing essential oils you'd like. Pour the mixture into the bath as it's filling up, just as you would bath salts.

MAKES ENOUGH FOR 1 OR 2 BATHS

INGREDIENTS

1 cup (240 ml) yogurt

1 cup (240 g) Epsom salts

INSTRUCTIONS

Combine both ingredients together; refrigerate until use.

SPIRULINA FACE MASK

Spa time is a lovely evening activity, so why not get clearer skin while you're at it? Bentonite clay is used as the main ingredient in many home-made face masks to detoxify skin, shrink pores, and treat acne. Cider vinegar, instead of water, helps the clay dissolve, while the cider vinegar itself kills acne-causing bacteria.

Why spirulina in this recipe? The chlorophyll in it cleans your skin,

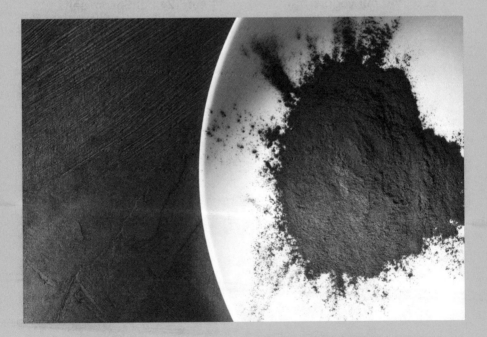

and, when used topically, spirulina can reduce redness and rosacea. Plus, it's good for cell turnover and faster healing, just in case you have any blemishes or marks you're currently staring at, wishing they'd settle down a little more quickly. This mask works best when applied before getting into a bath and washed off after, for a two-in-one self-care evening.

MAKES 1 FACE MASK

INGREDIENTS

1 tablespoon bentonite clay

½ teaspoon spirulina powder

1 tablespoon cider vinegar, or more if needed

INSTRUCTIONS

Combine all the ingredients into a spreadable consistency, adding more cider vinegar if needed. It should be the thickness of paste.

CHAMOMILE BATH SALTS

Without anything added for fragrance, bath salts are just, well, salts and some baking soda. When you buy them from bath shops, a big part of the appeal is how good they smell, and I think this recipe beats anything you can buy in the store when it comes to super good smells! And if by some chance you're a person who dislikes fragrance, just ditch the scent for your perfect bath.

No surprises here: chamomile and Epsom salts together make for a sleepy, good-smelling bath experience. Since Epsom salts are made of

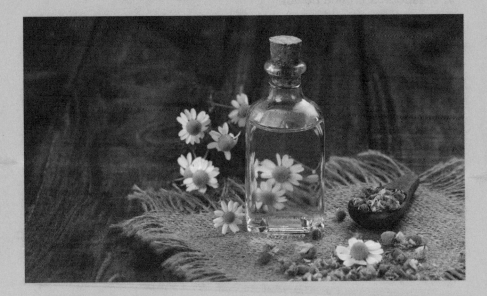

magnesium and not actual salt, you can add sea salt to this too, if you'd like. That will add the benefit of improving circulation and balancing your skin's moisture. I wanted to keep things as easy as possible, though. Baking soda detoxifies your body, as well as makes your skin softer. If you've been in a pool and are having a hard time feeling free of that unpleasant chlorine odor, baking soda can assist—it's known for its odor neutralization with good reason! And finally, the floral aroma of chamomile will help you relax before you even enter the tub. Add the salts as the tub is filling with water.

MAKES ENOUGH FOR 1 OR 2 BATHS

INGREDIENTS

1 cup (240 g) Epsom salts

¼ cup (45 g) baking soda

20 drops chamomile essential oil

INSTRUCTIONS

Combine all the ingredients in a bowl, and store in a tightly sealed jar or Tupperware.

LAVENDER BATH SCRUB

My goal here was to create a bath scrub that, after you've sufficiently scoured yourself clean, makes a great bath soak. Once you've filled your tub, you deserve to be able to enjoy yourself until the water has cooled! By using both the essential oil and flower itself, you get a double hit of lavender's soothing aroma benefits, plus the exfoliation from the plant matter and the beautiful look of the petals. Sea salt ups the exfoliating ante—it's also full of minerals that will help prevent your fingers and toes from getting prune-like, further facilitating this long-term bath relationship. Any neutral oil will do, but try to choose one that isn't GMO, which cheaper vegetable oils usually are. That said, no need to go spendy! Seed oils such as sunflower or grape seed work just fine here.

MAKES ENOUGH FOR 4 TO 6 BATHS

INGREDIENTS

20 drops lavender oil

1 tablespoon dried lavender flowers

½ cup (120 g) sea salt

⅓ cup (80 ml) neutral oil, such as sunflower or grape seed

INSTRUCTIONS

Combine all the ingredients in a bowl; store in a tightly sealed jar.

INDEX

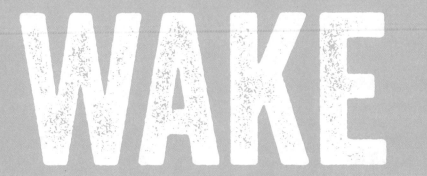

WAKE

WHAT TO EAT AND DO FOR MORE ENERGY

ARIANE RESNICK, CNC

The Countryman Press
A division of W. W. Norton & Company
Independent Publishers Since 1923

Copyright © 2019 by Ariane Resnick

For information about permission to
reproduce selections from this book, write
to Permissions, The Countryman Press,
500 Fifth Avenue, New York, NY 10110

For information about special discounts for
bulk purchases, please contact
W. W. Norton Special Sales at specialsales@
wwnorton.com or 800-233-4830

Manufacturing by Versa Press
Book design by Ashley Prine, Tandem Books
Production manager: Devon Zahn

The Countryman Press
www.countrymanpress.com

A division of W. W. Norton & Company, Inc.
500 Fifth Avenue, New York, NY 10110
www.wwnorton.com

978-1-68268-321-7 (pbk.)

10 9 8 7 6 5 4 3 2 1

CONTENTS

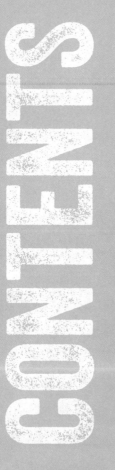

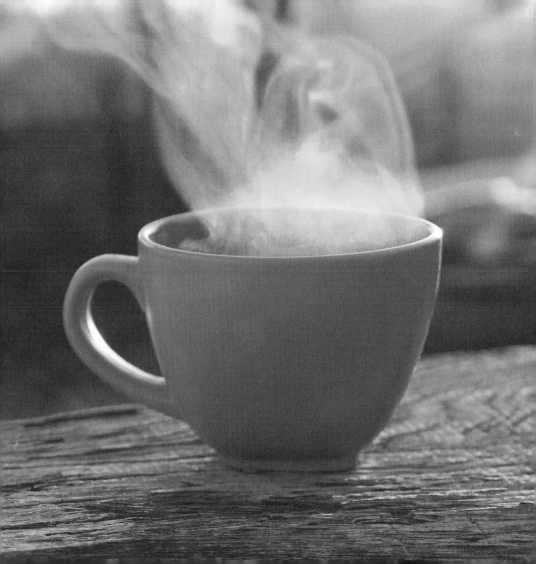

INTRODUCTION

WHAT IS CAFFEINE, WHAT DOES IT DO, AND WHY ARE WE SO HOOKED ON IT?

GOOD MORNING!

IF YOU'RE ANYTHING LIKE 90 PERCENT OF THE POPULATION OF the United States, your day begins with a caffeinated beverage. Caffeine helps us wake up, but that's only the beginning of its many benefits. Numerous scientific studies have revealed that caffeine enhances mood, improves focus, increases muscle stamina, and prevents weight gain. Beyond that, there is even evidence that caffeine can decrease chronic inflammation, stimulate hair growth, reduce risk (and symptoms) of fatty liver, ward off Alzheimer's disease, and even increase sperm count.

Our love of this stimulant isn't anything new, either. To cite just a few examples of our age-old crush on caffeine: the consumption of tea dates back nearly five thousand years; the leaves of the coffee plant were used medicinally in Africa in the 1100s; and ancient Maya drank cocoa as a part of their wedding rituals. The

Wake portion of this book is devoted to our enduring love of caffeine, with 26 food, bevvie, and DIY recipes that will really perk up your mornings. As a certified nutritionist known for my wellness work, it's incredibly important to me that these recipes also contribute to your health, rather than take away from it.

The Technical Stuff

Caffeine is a chemical compound that stimulates your brain and central nervous system. It helps you stay alert by blocking the effects of adenosine, the neurotransmitter that makes you feel sleepy. Adenosine is produced when your body uses up

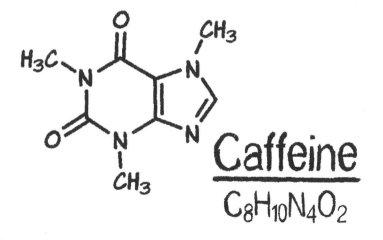

Caffeine
$$C_8H_{10}N_4O_2$$

its supply of adenosine triphosphate (ATP), the chemical compound needed for cellular energy. When you stop adenosine from being effective, you stop the subsequent sleepiness that would otherwise ensue. Because of the way caffeine antagonizes the adenosine receptors, it has been studied for potential use in treatments for illnesses such as Parkinson's and epilepsy. It does this through its neuroprotective properties, meaning that blocking adenosine can slow down, stop, or even reverse negative changes in your nervous system, as well as help to manage motor deficits.

What Is Caffeinated?

As you probably already know, caffeinated foods and beverages include tea, coffee, and chocolate; but did you know it's also in kombucha? There are countless ways to enjoy caffeine beyond just brewing some tea or cocoa. A cup of morning joe or a mug of your favorite tea is unarguably a great thing, but half the fun of life is in switching things up! Because caffeine is used so functionally, most people don't think about the fact that there is so much more that can be done with caffeine beyond however we take our usual cup. This book will not only look in depth at the caffeinated foods and drinks we know and love, it will offer new and interesting ways to use them. There are plenty of additional plants with stimulating effects, such as kola nut, guarana, and blackbrush,

but they can be a bit hard to come by, so we'll stick to the simple options. We want waking up to be easier, not more complex.

Wake Recipes

To make sure you're truly motivated to take this book right into the kitchen with you, all the recipes I've provided are lightning fast—or at least moderately quick—to make. They can also be created without chef-level culinary skills or access to elite ingredients. I believe in focusing on whole foods that can be found at neighborhood grocers, with methods that rely on adding flavor by way of quality ingredients. That's why all my Wake recipes are organized around a few readily available, whole-food ingredients: coffee, kombucha, tea, and cocoa. My motto is that eating and drinking well can, and should, be joyful, and there is no easier way to put that motto to good use than with an ingredient selection that naturally brings joy!

I'm an advocate of caffeinated food and drink because caffeine has so many health benefits. It also just plain makes you feel good, which counts for a lot. However, that doesn't mean every preparation of a caffeinated item is an intelligent one. I'm looking at you, syrup-laden mocha frappuccinos made with factory-farmed milk and corn syrup. Any caffeinated drink or treat from a mainstream cafe that tastes too good to be good for you probably is *not* good for you—even if it is matcha green and has a healthy sounding name.

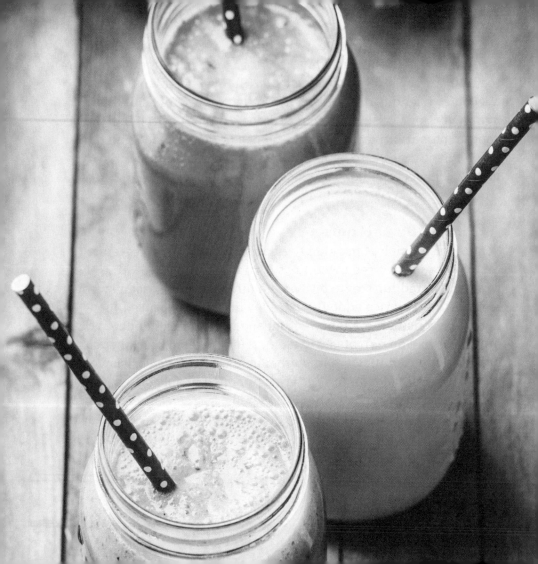

As is my signature style, the recipes in this book are all gluten-free, can easily be made sugar-free (if they aren't already), and are focused on whole-food ingredients. With few exceptions, they're also paleo friendly, grain-free, and either vegan or come with a vegan version. I also never use starches, gums, or products that contain preservatives, because who needs 'em? It's amazing how much flavor there is to be found in single ingredients, and how much delicious buzz you can add to your day!

A Note on Sweeteners

Wherever possible, I provide the option for you to "sweeten to taste" because desired sweetness is so individual. In testing these recipes, I opted for stevia or Swerve (an erythritol-based sweetener with prebiotics added) wherever possible, because I just don't like consuming a lot of actual sugar or recommending that others do so. You can also use monk fruit, a.k.a. lo han, though I don't tend to find it sweet enough. Some naturally caloric sweeteners are used, mostly in the forms of honey, maple syrup, and coconut sugar, and when they are liquid, the recipes require that quantity of liquid. Feel free to experiment with combos of caloric and non-caloric sweeteners that best serve your own health and taste buds!

Fabulous Fats

In baked goods, unless butter is being used, I typically call for a "neutral" oil. This means a cooking oil that doesn't have any inherent flavor of its own. (An example of a non-neutral oil would be olive oil, which has a strong taste.) There are countless neutral cooking oils on the market, some of which are healthier than others. I recommend avoiding low-quality oils, such as generic "vegetable" oil or sunflower oil, as these are high in inflammatory omega-6 fatty acids. Instead, opt for grape seed oil as your cheapest option, or avocado oil if your budget allows for it.

The Fine Print

You know your body best. Chances are that if you picked up this book, you enjoy caffeinated foods and are excited to use them in inventive, new ways. However, if you're sensitive to caffeine, make sure you only choose the recipes that use less-caffeinated items, such as kombucha, or try first playing around in the DIY chapter, which features pick-me-ups that are not ingested. If you have any health issues that make caffeine questionable for you, check into that thoroughly with your medical professional before trying any recipes.

Always listen to your body to make sure you're comfortable

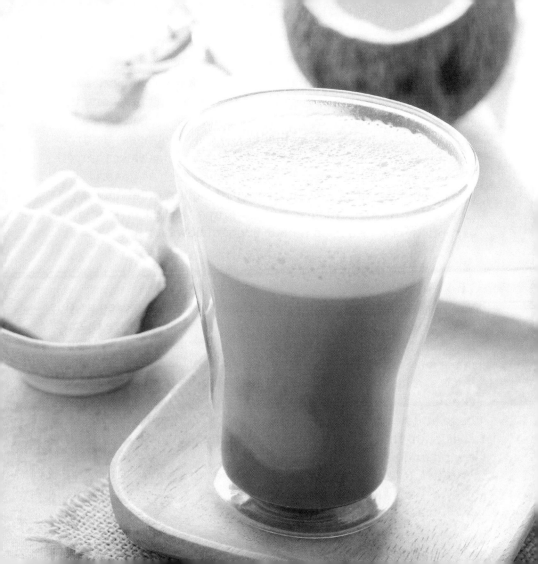

with caffeine's effects. If you find yourself too caffeinated because you tried too many *Wake* recipes, all you have to do is flip over to the *Sleep* side of this book for recipes to help you chill back out!

DIY Wake: Beyond Caffeine

While caffeine definitely has the market cornered for everyday stimulants, there are other useful ingredients that need not be eaten to put some serious pep in your step. For weekends or other times when you're able to start your morning a bit more leisurely, I've provided some simple DIY projects that will help widen your eyes and bush up your tail. Eucalyptus, for example, is an invigorating plant with a smell that goes deep into your sinuses, so we'll make a shower spray that's perfect for times you need an extra boost in your morning ritual. Bonus: It can also help you feel better if you're having any cold symptoms! Citrus oils lift mood and improve your complexion, so we'll make a toning spritz that provides both benefits.

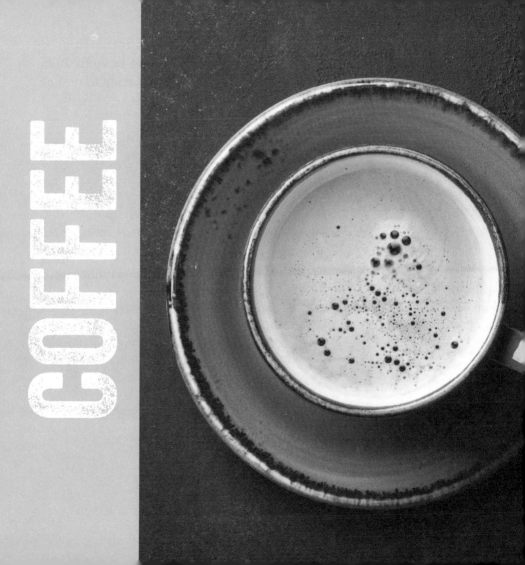
COFFEE

REALLY, IT'S GOOD FOR YOU!

Perhaps, like me, you've had periods in your life when you gave up coffee because you considered it a guilty pleasure. Sure, it makes you feel like you can take over the world, but some health and wellness folks claim you're basically ruining yourself, your adrenals, and your life by drinking it. It's only in recent years that science has gotten on board with what most of us coffee drinkers have long suspected: this scrumptious bean actually is good for you.

While caffeine used to be considered carcinogenic by the World Health Organization, in 2016 (thanks to multitudinous studies) the organization did an about-face and placed it on the cancer-*preventative* list. Nowadays, coffee drinking is recognized for its association with longer life spans, lower rates of diabetes, and reduced rates of multiple types of cancer. Coffee can even prevent Alzheimer's, with studies showing as much as a 65 percent reduced risk of the disease! Coffee contains antioxidants and has an assortment of B vitamins; a single cup offers more than 10 percent of the recommended dietary allowance (RDA) for vitamin B2 and 6 percent of the RDA for B5.

Get the Most Out of It

How much coffee is beneficial to your health? It's generally recommended that you don't consume more than three to four cups a day, as that can lead to poor sleep quality and increased blood pressure. For most people, that's double their average daily consumption, so no worries there. One serving of the majority of the Wake recipes is equivalent to about one-eighth to one full cup of coffee, so keep that in mind when you're gassing up in the morning.

If you experience any of coffee's potential negative effects, such as jitters or nervousness, you're probably better off drinking or eating it with fat, such as butter (it's called "Bulletproof," and trust me, it's delicious; see page 34.) or heavy cream, which slows down your body's absorption of the caffeine. Having caffeine with fat leads to a longer-lasting, smoother buzz with less comedown later. Bulletproof in Bed Coffee and Golden Glow Turmeric Latte are great slow-burn Wake recipes that will keep you charged up for a long time. Just be careful that you don't have a fat-filled coffee item too late in the day, as it could keep you up at night because the caffeine wears off more slowly.

If you have issues with the acidity, try a coffee with reduced acid content (there are many on the market now that specifically contain less acid) and/or opt for a brewing method that reduces acidity, such as pour-overs or cold brew.

The Yum Factor

In addition to its varied health benefits, the taste of coffee is an easy one to work with. No matter the varietal, it's a rich, deep, and robust food, and it holds up well to other flavors being added to it, from standard baking ingredients such as vanilla and cinnamon to fruits such as bananas and berries. Whether you take your morning cup in a protein shake or hot and black, you're bound to resonate with these recipes that play on standard flavors as well as new, more unusual ones.

TYPES OF COFFEE

French, Italian, Sumatra, or a blend of 10 other types: what coffee itself *should* taste like is completely up to you. Some prefer a light, fruity African bean that's scarcely heavier than tea, while others want a New York style "cup of mud." Personally, I love a heavy, dark roast, and I strongly favor coffee blends with chicory added. These rec-

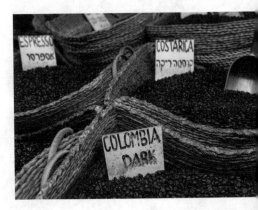

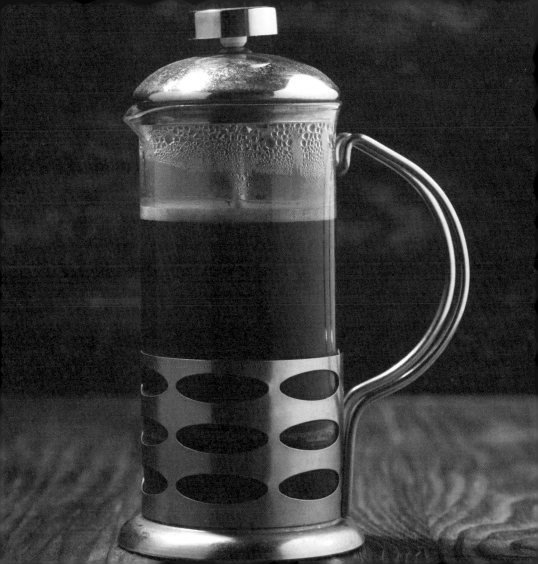

ipes were tested with multiple types of coffee to ensure that no matter what you have in the cabinet, you'll get a delicious result.

BREWING METHODS

The following are common ways of preparing coffee. Where it's important to use a particular method for a recipe, I've specified which I recommend. Otherwise, choose your favorite brewing method. (I'm skipping the niche options such as Chemex and Aeropress, because if you do have them, you're probably a bit of a coffee aficionado and already have their basics down pat!)

DRIP: This is the most common method for brewing coffee. Standard coffeemakers produce what is known as drip coffee, and they do so by the potful. You add a filter, coffee, and water, and the machine does the rest. This method involves plastic getting heated, which can offset the flavor of your coffee, and you can't control the temperature of the water.

FRENCH PRESS: My personal favorite method, French presses come in sizes from single cup and up, and they allow you to control the water temp completely. Simply pour in coffee grounds and hot water, then stir and place the lid on top until it's ready, at which time you press down so the grounds get trapped under the liquid.

You can also decide on the strength of your coffee based on how long you let it brew. Unless otherwise noted, the recipes in this chapter were tested with French-pressed coffee, which I brewed for about 10 minutes.

KEURIG/NESPRESSO/SINGLE-SERVE MACHINES: In general, I make a point of being a nondogmatic person who judges as little as possible. Please keep that in mind right now as I emphatically implore you to just say no to these things! Outside of the immense and tragic environmental impact of a bazillion tiny plastic pods, this is a guaranteed way to produce the worst-tasting cup of coffee possible. Sure, it's a minute faster, but how many minutes will you suffer through that lousy-tasting cup for?

POUR-OVER: Made popular by the "coffee 2.0" or "new wave" coffee movements of the last decade, as artisan coffeehouses became commonplace across the country, pour-overs involve streaming water over your ground beans in a filtered device directly into a cup. This releases most of the acidity into the air, making for an incredibly smooth coffee. On the downside, if you're a fan of strong coffee, you might find it too mild.

ESPRESSO: I initially used a stovetop espresso maker for the espresso-based Wake recipes. This is a convenient contraption in which you place grounds and water. You heat it on the stove,

and you get a cup that's definitely stronger than standard coffee. Even so, I didn't feel that it had the heaviness or thickness that I expected out of espresso, so I ended up having my sous chef order a big mug of espresso from the shop down the street so that we could retest using that. If you have a countertop home espresso maker, your results will be more similar to cafe style than the stovetop version. This is preferred, if possible, but a stovetop maker will work in a pinch.

COLD BREW: This easy way of brewing coffee takes some patience . . . typically about 16 hours' worth. You add coffee to cold water at a high concentrated proportion, such as a ratio of 1 cup (240 ml) coffee to 4 cups (960 ml) water, then let it sit at least overnight before straining. Typically, cold brew is then mixed 1:1 with water or ice for serving. The concentrate lasts a week or two in the fridge, so it's an awesome choice for summer imbibing.

RECIPES

GOLDEN GLOW TURMERIC LATTE

It's not nearly as well-known as it should be that coffee is an anti-inflammatory food. It is, on the other hand, very well-known that turmeric is. What happens when you combine the two elements? You get a soothing yet energizing beverage that contributes to your wellness rather than detracts from it. By adding coconut butter, you get a rich mouthfeel that helps balance the bite of turmeric; a burst of medium-chain fatty acids, which boost metabolism; plus a dose of immune-enhancing lauric acid. Because turmeric is fat-soluble, consuming it with the fat of coconut butter and heavy cream may help you reap its benefits more completely than having it as a tea alone. This concept is Bulletproof-esque (see page 34), making it a cut above your average turmeric drink. It's also more filling than one without fats, which is an extra plus if you drink caffeine to curb your appetite.

MAKES 1 SERVING

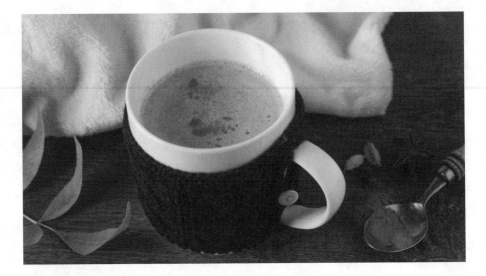

INGREDIENTS

1 cup (240 ml) hot coffee

1½ teaspoons coconut butter

1½ teaspoons heavy cream or coconut creamer

½ teaspoon turmeric powder (or more if you're cool with the taste)

Stevia or maple syrup to taste

INSTRUCTIONS

In a small pot over low heat, mix all the ingredients until the turmeric powder and coconut butter are thoroughly incorporated.

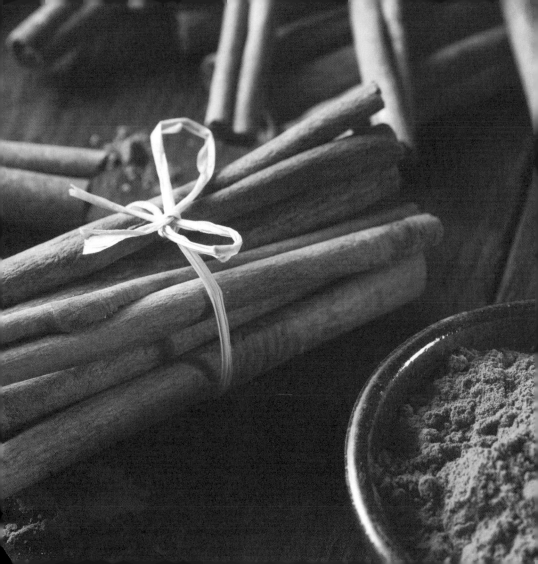

HOT-CHATA LATTE

Horchata is a milky, sweet, and thick Spanish beverage that is tradition-ally made without any actual milk. You soak rice or nuts overnight, then blend in sweetener, cinnamon, and vanilla, then strain. Because I don't want you to have to think about your latte the night before, this simpli-fied version is instead made with the nut or rice milk of your choice. I add heavy cream or coconut creamer for thickness, as a nondairy milk alone won't give you the rich texture of horchata. I also favor espresso over coffee, so the drink doesn't get watered down. It is made stovetop so you don't need the blender and, unlike a traditional horchata recipe, it doesn't require any straining.

MAKES 1 SERVING

INGREDIENTS

1 large shot espresso (2–3 tablespoons)

¾ cup (180 ml) almond or rice milk (or other milk of your choice)

1 tablespoon heavy cream

¼ teaspoon cinnamon

½ teaspoon vanilla

Stevia or maple syrup to taste

INSTRUCTIONS

1. In a small pot over medium-low heat, combine all the ingredients.

2. Stir to incorporate the cinnamon thoroughly and heat until very lightly steaming.

COFFEE COFFEE CAKE

Coffee cake is already delish on its own or eaten with a cup of coffee, but what if you add the coffee right into the cake for a two-for experience? You get something that I gave myself a major pat on the back for having come up with, and I trust you'll enjoy it as much as I do. Sure, I didn't invent it (internet searches do indeed yield a few results), but I do believe this is the healthiest one out there! Also, others use instant coffee, which I give a major thumbs-down to when it comes to taste. Instead, I use espresso, which you don't even need to brew right when you make the cake. If it's easier for you to buy it and store it in the fridge for a day or two, that works perfectly well. To give this recipe a more classic texture, there's an optional streusel topping. I think the cake is rich enough without it, but streusel certainly doesn't ever hurt things!

MAKES 8 LARGE OR 12 SMALL SERVINGS

INGREDIENTS

DRY

1½ cups (175 g) almond flour

½ cup (60 g) coconut flour

½ cup (100 g) Swerve or cane sugar, or a combo

1 teaspoon baking soda

1 teaspoon cinnamon

½ teaspoon salt

WET

¼ cup (60 ml, or 2–3 large shots) espresso

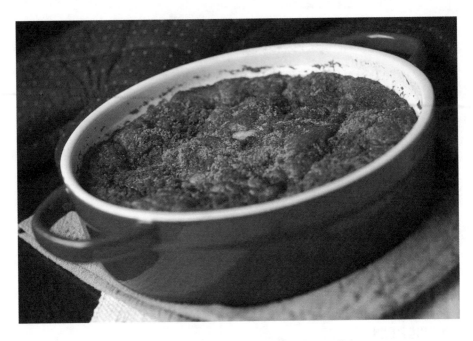

3 eggs or vegan egg replacer equivalent

½ cup (120 ml) neutral oil, such as avocado or grape seed

¼ cup (60 ml) Greek yogurt (dairy or coconut)

¼ cup (60 ml) honey

1 teaspoon vanilla extract

1 teaspoon coffee extract, optional

INSTRUCTIONS

1. Preheat the oven to 350°F (175°C).

2. In a large mixing bowl, combine all the dry ingredients with a fork or whisk, making sure no lumps of almond or coconut flour remain.

3. Add all the wet ingredients to the dry and stir until uniform in texture.

4. Pour the batter into a greased 9-inch (23 cm) cake pan, add optional topping if desired (see below), and bake about 30 minutes, or until a knife inserted comes out clean.

OPTIONAL TOPPING INGREDIENTS

¼ cup (55 g) salted butter

½ cup (60 g) almond flour

½ cup (100 g) sugar (coconut, cane, or a combo)

2 tablespoons coconut flour

Large pinch cinnamon

INSTRUCTIONS

Pulse all the ingredients together in a food processor until crumbly, or combine by hand with a pastry blender.

COFFEE-FLOUR SPICE COOKIES

So, coffee flour . . . it's not exactly the dream of an ingredient it sounds like. Sure, it looks just how you'd imagine: dark brown and feathery light. But the taste? This stuff is made from the coffee cherry, a.k.a. the fruit of the plant that usually gets discarded, not from the bean itself. As such, coffee flour is great for the environment (yay, less waste!), but it's not exactly delectable on its own, nor does its taste resemble coffee beans in any way. It took me a few tries to come up with a recipe I love, as its sour and bitter characteristics overpowered other ingredients unless I barely used any, which defeated the purpose. It was worth the effort, though, because these cookies are scrumptious! The spices pair well with the coffee flour's taste—I don't recommend making this recipe without them.

Coffee flour has about the same amount of caffeine as chocolate, meaning these cookies will give you a little zing.

MAKES 12–16 COOKIES

INGREDIENTS

- 1 cup (240 ml) nut butter (I used peanut)
- 1 cup (100 g) sugar, Swerve, monk fruit, or a combo
- 2 eggs
- 3 tablespoons coffee flour
- 1½ teaspoons cinnamon
- 1 teaspoon baking soda
- ½ teaspoon ginger
- ¼ teaspoon salt
- Pinch cloves

BULLETPROOF IN BED COFFEE

Bulletproof coffee is something I've been a fan of for a super long time. Its silky, sexy texture comes from blending delectable butter and brain-boosting MCT oil into each cup. (*MCT* means "medium chain triglycerides," a form of fat that bypasses the liver for processing and goes straight to your brain for fuel.) I use the Bulletproof brand called Brain Octane Oil, because it is highly concentrated, as well as fairly traded and free of rainforest-harming palm oil. Since I can't leave well enough alone, I craft Bulletproof coffee with adaptogenic herbs, grass-fed beef gelatin (a form of collagen created through cooking), and other health-boosting ingredients, and this recipe is my all-time favorite version.

If you have concerns about coffee harming your adrenal glands, this is a surefire way to mitigate that issue. Maca is one adaptogenic herb I can't shut up about. It boosts your sex drive, regulates your hormones, and even increases breast milk production. I prefer versions made with the fiber taken out to avoid potential bloating.

MAKES 1 SERVING

INGREDIENTS

1 cup (240 ml) hot coffee

1 tablespoon Brain Octane Oil

1 tablespoon grass-fed butter (I prefer cultured, salted butter)

1 teaspoon maca powder

Stevia to taste, optional

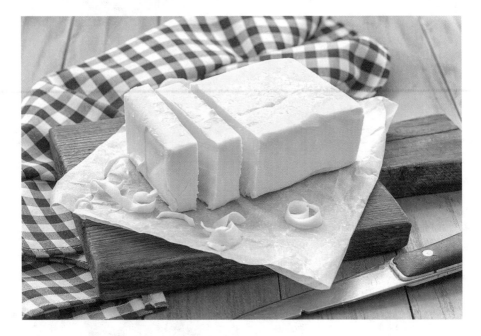

INSTRUCTIONS

In a blender, combine all the ingredients until creamy and frothy.

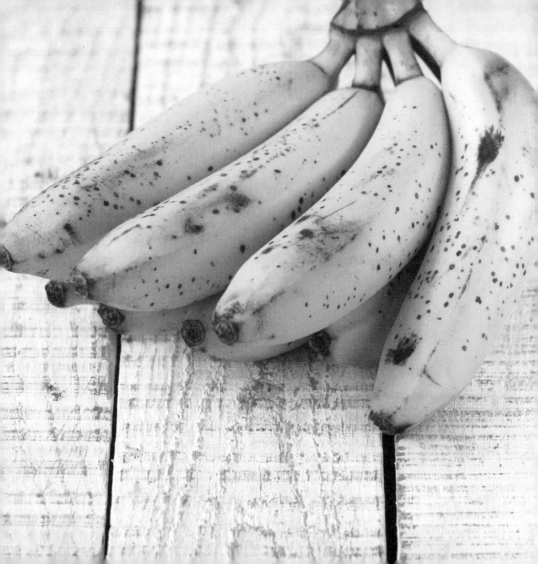

NANA MOCHA PROTEIN POPS

There is literally no quicker way to take homemade coffee on the go than to pull a popsicle or two out of the freezer. The protein powder and mineral-rich bananas in these pops make them a solid breakfast or an afternoon pick-me-up treat. The cocoa powder lends a great chocolaty taste and adds fiber without adding sugar. If you want to make these extra dessert-y, swap the cocoa out for a few tablespoons of chocolate chips, or add them in addition to the cocoa powder if you are a chocolate fiend (which I have mad respect for, and can definitely relate to).

MAKES 8 STANDARD-SIZE POPSICLES OR 12 SMALL ONES

INGREDIENTS

2 cups (480 ml) cold-brew coffee (see page 23; or use refrigerated, regularly brewed coffee if this sounds like too much effort)

2 scoops protein powder (I use vanilla bone broth protein)

1 cup (150 g) very ripe, frozen banana pieces (about 1 small banana)

2 tablespoons cocoa powder

INSTRUCTIONS

1. In a blender, combine all the ingredients until smooth.

2. Pour into popsicle molds and freeze for 3 to 4 hours or until solid.

COLLAGEN COFFEE SHAKE

Collagen is one of those buzzwords that just won't quit. The product came into popular use and has stayed there because those who use it tend to notice benefits such as stronger nails, faster-growing hair, and less-wrinkled skin. It's also easy to add to your food, as it's a tasteless powder that dissolves in liquids without any grit or residue. In addition to adding collagen to meals, eating foods that promote collagen production is also important. Vitamin C plays a vital role in helping your body produce collagen, so say "Yes, please" to berries and other C-rich foods. When it comes to coffee, I go with raspberries because the flavors and colors combine so well.

MAKES 1 SERVING

INGREDIENTS

¾ cup (180 ml) cold-brew coffee (see page 23; or use refrigerated, regularly brewed coffee if this sounds like too much effort)

½ cup (70 g) frozen raspberries

½ cup (70 g) ice

¼ cup (60 ml) vanilla yogurt (dairy or non)

1 teaspoon honey, or more to taste

1 serving collagen powder

INSTRUCTIONS

In a blender, combine all the ingredients until thick and creamy.

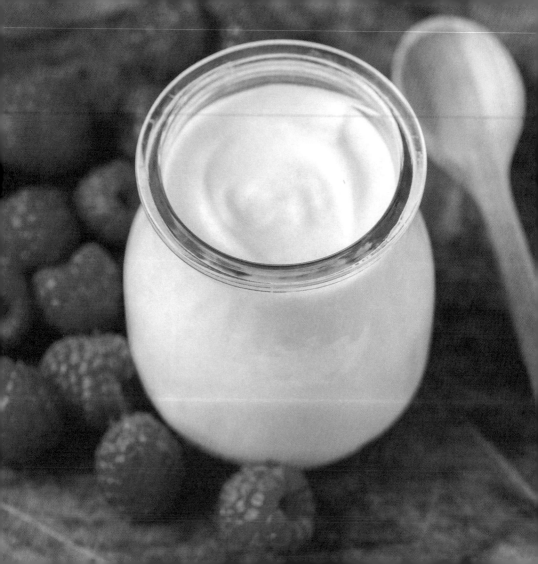

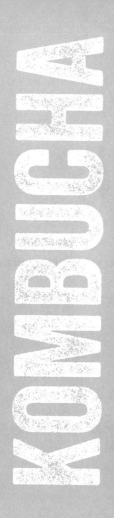

KOMBUCHA

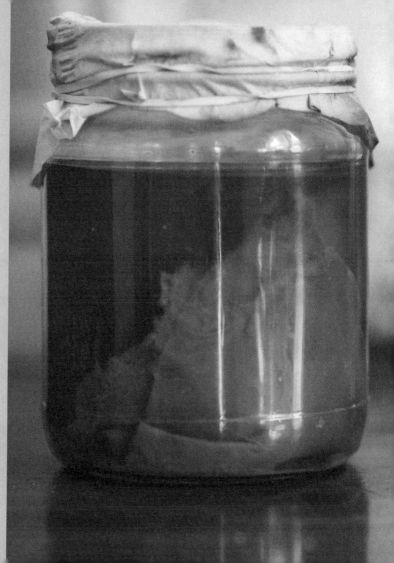

HOW IT CAME TO FAME

Nearly a decade ago, a down-and-out movie star brought kombucha into the pop-culture limelight when her home-arrest alcohol-sensor bracelet went off. Lindsay Lohan hadn't been drinking booze, but rather, a fizzy fermented beverage said to cure everything from digestive issues to cancer. Suddenly, kombucha was pulled from the shelves of health food stores across the country, and brands had to begin testing for alcohol content.

When kombucha returned to the market, some brands' bottles declared minimal alcohol contents that could be bought by consumers of any age, and others touted alcohol contents high enough to require imbibers be 21 years or older to purchase them. Whether under or over the legal limit, our culture was suddenly aware of this ages-old cultured drink, and it took off. Today, there are countless brands available in stores both health food and mainstream, and the drink can even be found at gas stations. Kombucha fans love it for its digestive properties and the mild buzz it gives you. Though some of the caffeine is

eaten up in the fermentation process (more on that below), it still provides a solid amount of pick-me-up.

So WTF Is It?

Kombucha isn't anything new. It's been around for at least a couple thousand years, dating back to ancient China, where it was used as a health tonic. It's a fermented beverage made by combining brewed tea with sugar and a strange thing called a SCOBY, which stands for "symbiotic culture of bacteria and yeast." The SCOBY eats the sugar and creates probiotics in turn. After about a month of countertop fermentation, what was once sweet tea becomes a probiotic, lightly carbonated drink with a tangy taste somewhat similar to vinegar.

Are the Health Claims Real?

Some of the claims about kombucha's health benefits have been substantiated through studies, but not all. The ones that have been proven scientifically are:

PROBIOTICS: Kombucha contains multiple strains of probiotics, which are well proven to improve gut health and immunity.

ANTI ASSORTED BAD BUGS: Studies have shown kombucha to be antimicrobial and antibacterial, as well as antagonizing to candida (mean-

ing it attacks all the bad bugs in your gut). While probiotics are good bugs that you need, they aren't necessarily strong enough to kill off all bad ones, so some extra fighting power is helpful!

POLYPHENOLS: It retains the polyphenols of the tea it is made from, which means it also retains the health benefits of the green, black, white, or whatever tea was used to make the kombucha in question. Learn more about tea's benefits in the tea chapter (page 54)!

Should I Make It Myself?

You certainly can if you'd like to! That's a project I'm not going to get into here, as personally I haven't had great luck with it, and this book is about quick recipes rather than 30-day ones. My experience is that making your own kombucha does not exactly yield the same yummy drink you can buy. It is, however, much more cost effective. If you're inspired to brew your own, *The Big Book of Kombucha* by Hannah Crum and Alex LaGory has everything you need to know.

The Flavor Spectrum

Once a niche market, the world of kombucha has grown to a practically endless flavor spectrum made available by countless brands. I recommend choosing drinks with a lower sugar content; other-

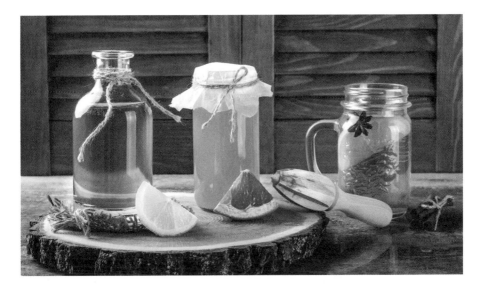

wise you defeat the effects of probiotics for gut wellness. Also, high sugar is indicative of a milder 'booch that likely won't offer the same health benefits or buzz as a stronger, low-sugar option.

A Nod to Jun

Making its way into major health food chains is a version of kombucha made with honey instead of sugar, known as jun. The result of using a different sweetener doesn't seem like it would be important, but if you ask me, jun tastes even better than kombucha does.

The only reason I didn't use it in the recipes in this chapter is because it isn't widely available for purchase yet. But if you can find it, by all means, swap out the kombucha in any recipe for your favorite flavor of jun.

The Importance of Caffeine

Kombucha expert Hannah Crum says kombucha must be brewed in caffeinated tea because "brewing with the tea plant, *Camellia Sinensis*, is a vital part of a continuing, healthy kombucha batch after batch. This is due to the many components present, including naturally occurring caffeine. Just like humans, yeasts feature nervous systems that are triggered by caffeine. In kombucha fermentation, caffeine spurs the yeast into action, quickly lowering the pH before mold can grow on the sweet tea. As it is consumed by the brewing process, the remaining caffeine is usually less than one-third the amount in a typical cup of tea."

Keeping the Probiotics Alive

Because kombucha contains probiotics, which are literally alive, it's important that you don't cook it if you want to reap the benefits of the good bugs. Because of that, most of these recipes require no heat at all. Where kombucha is heated, only part of it is, and it does not need to be boiled.

RECIPES

SINGLE-FRUIT SLUSHIE

This recipe couldn't be any simpler, but boy does it taste like you spent some quality time on it! The ratio can be used for basically any type of kombucha with any frozen fruit, and the end result will still be a fizzy slushie that drinks as if it has far more than two ingredients. The boost of probiotics is especially helpful since fruit can be yeast-promoting. Why not cut down on your candida worries with a frosty bevvie?!

The favorite taste-tested combo was frozen mango with strawberry kombucha, which is basically summertime through a straw. Other hits were grape kombucha plus blackberries or raspberries, ginger kombucha plus pineapple, or citrus kombucha with watermelon.

MAKES 1 SERVING

INGREDIENTS

1 cup (240 ml) kombucha (flavored or not, per your preference)

1 cup (150 g) frozen fruit (a single fruit or a combination)

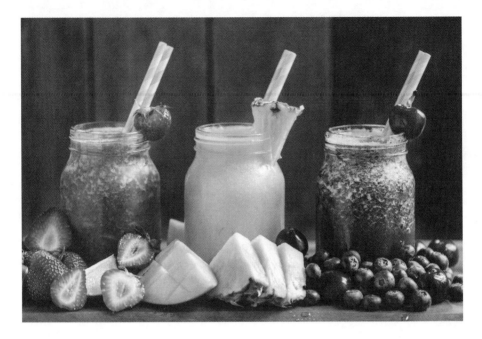

INSTRUCTIONS

In a blender, combine all the ingredients until uniform in texture.

BE JELLY OF THE GELLY CANDIES

Kombucha gummies are a staple of the paleo food world, as the gut-healing combination of grass-fed gelatin and kombucha is a powerful one. Typically the goal is for these gummies to be as firm as possible so that you can take them on the go. This recipe, however, is more of a dessert or snack that you can still eat with your hands but has a little bit of a softer and more jelly-like texture. What's the fun in life without variety?! If you want to make these more like traditional gummies, just add an additional tablespoon or two of gelatin.

Similar to the slushie recipe, you can use any fruit combined with any kombucha—what matters most is that you've pureed the fruit, so that it's smooth with no bits and pieces. Since you won't be heating most of the kombucha, don't stress about heating it too much. As far as molds go, silicone is the easiest to work with. Choose large or small shapes, whichever you prefer; the selection on the internet or craft stores is pretty huge! If using a pan, glass is easiest to slice or cookie-cut them out of.

MAKES 12 SERVINGS

INGREDIENTS

1½ cups (360 ml) kombucha (flavored or not, per your preference)

½ cup (120 ml) cold water

¼ cup (35 g) powdered gelatin

1 cup (240 ml) fruit puree

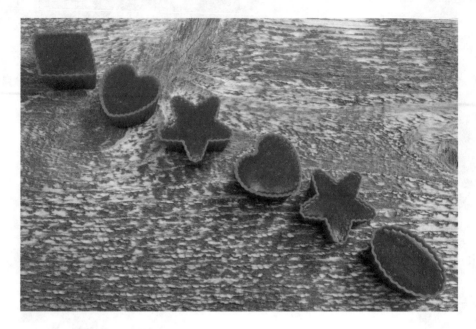

INSTRUCTIONS

1. In a saucepan, combine ½ cup (120 ml) of the kombucha with the cold water and sprinkle the gelatin over top. Let it bloom for about 5 minutes.

2. Heat the mixture over low heat until glossy, with no gelatin lumps; take moderate care not to overheat, which will kill the probiotics in the kombucha.

3. Remove from the heat and add the remaining kombucha and fruit puree, stirring until combined, then pour into a pan or molds and refrigerate until firm, 2 to 4 hours.

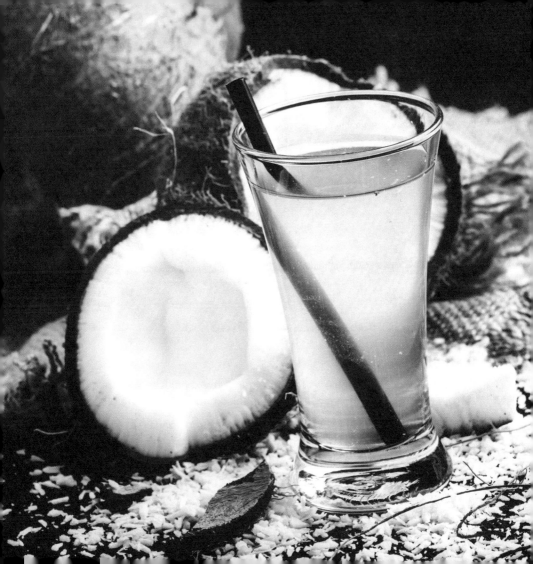

COCO-BUCHA SODA

Coconut water is inherently sweet and contains a great balance of electrolytes. It also has fiber and protein, making it pretty powerful for just being the water found naturally inside a produce item. When you add coconut water to kombucha, you succeed in mellowing out the harsh vinegar tang that makes most people who aren't fans of kombucha squinch up their faces in distaste over. You can use any flavor of kombucha for this incredibly simple recipe. Since it has a fun, light quality, I suggest you use family-friendly flavors such as grape, berry, or apple. For coconut water, I recommend any fresh, refrigerated brand over a shelf-stable one, as those taste much better.

MAKES 1 SERVING

INGREDIENTS

½ cup (120 ml) kombucha (flavored or not, per your preference)

½ cup (120 ml) coconut water

INSTRUCTIONS

Fill a glass with ice, then add the kombucha and coconut water.

KOMBUCHA MARY

Because "Bloody Kombucha" just does not have a good ring, may I present everyone's favorite brunch girl, the Bloody Mary, done sans booze . . . but not quite virgin, because you'll still get that kombucha buzz, and hey, it's probably noon anyway. The spices in a Bloody help to rev up your metabolism, which kombucha already has a positive impact on due to its caffeine, B vitamins, and chromium. Feel free to garnish this with enough shrubbery to call it a snack, and don't feel guilty like you might when imbibing vodka in the morning.

INGREDIENTS

½ cup (120 ml) plain kombucha

¼ cup (60 ml) tomato juice

2–3 dashes hot sauce, to taste

½ teaspoon horseradish

1 dash cracked black pepper

1 dash celery salt

2 dashes coconut aminos or Worcestershire sauce

Celery, pickles, and other veggies, for garnish

INSTRUCTIONS

1. Combine all ingredients except the veggies in a pint glass and stir (because kombucha is carbonated, I don't recommend shaking).

2. Add ice to fill and stir again, then garnish with celery, pickles, or other veggies.

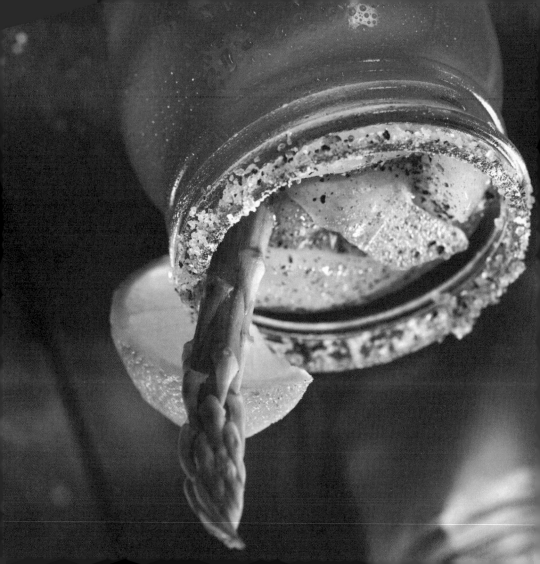

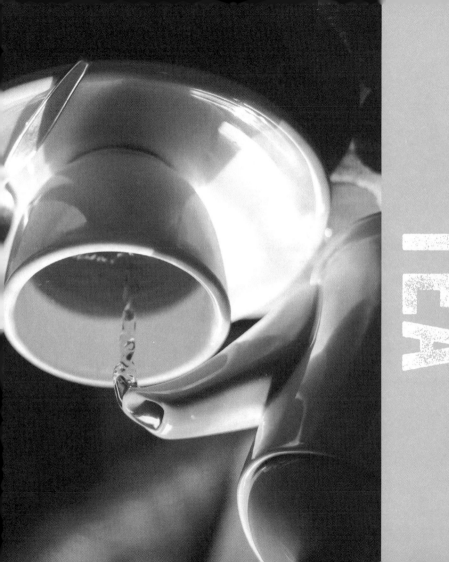

TEA

WHO HAS TIME FOR TEA TIME?

In America, coffee takes the morning cake, but in much of the rest of the world, tea is considered the premiere breakfast sipper. In fact, after water, it's the most-drunk drink in the world. Tea's caffeine content is lower than coffee, ranging from about 25 to 50 milligrams per cup. Originally cultivated in Asia, tea is made from the *Camellia Sinensis* plant and, with the exception of matcha (which we'll discuss more in a moment), is made by pouring boiling water over the plant's leaves. The leaves are then strained out, and the infused water is consumed as tea. As a country, China gulps down the most tea annually, but the residents of Turkey, Ireland, and the U.K. drink the most per person, with Turks brewing up an amazing 6.9 pounds (3 kg) on average each, annually.

What's the Buzz

Tea is nothing new, but its health benefits have been increasingly recognized in recent years. Of course tea

gives you all the perks of caffeine—including increased focus and a longer life span—but it is also full of antioxidant compounds. The most well-known group of antioxidants found in tea is polyphenols, and of those, tea is most known for a type called catechins. To go even further, of the catechins, tea is famous for its abundant EGCG (epigallocatechin gallate) content. What does all this mean? Tea is full of good stuff that helps you! In short, antioxidants do pretty much what their name promises—inhibit oxidation (think rust and corrosion). Antioxidants travel through your body canceling out some of the harm and wear that life has done to it. They protect you, to a limited extent, from heart problems, cancer, and general aging issues. You can even place tea bags over your eyes for the caffeine to aid in reducing puffiness!

Beyond the Cup

While tea is most commonly consumed as a beverage, just like coffee, its uses can extend far beyond that simple habit! Brewed tea is a great low-calorie base for desserts such as granitas and popsicles, and it pairs well with everything from orange juice to vanilla. The tea recipes in this chapter don't involve more work than simple brewing, but tea is also excellent for smoking foods, as it imparts a woody, milky aroma.

GIDGETS & GADGETS

Thanks to tea being so darned popular, the accessories you can buy to enhance your tea-drinking experience are quite varied. Even buying tea can be complex, with entire stores dedicated to it and its accoutrements. If you want to keep things simple, pour nearly boiling water over a bag of tea in a mug. If you want to get fancy, buy loose-leaf tea, put it into a tea ball or reusable netting, and steep it in a teapot. I didn't want

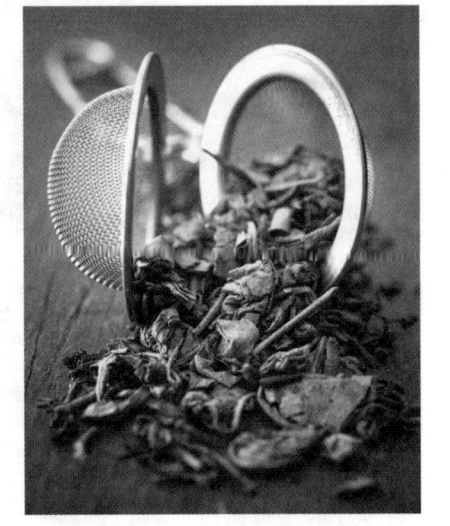

to assume you'd be so into tea that you'd do the latter, so I created these recipes with pre-bagged tea and no pots. As someone more into coffee than tea, that's my personal go-to method.

TYPES OF TEA

BLACK: The most common varietals of tea are black teas. Iced tea and other non-specific tea beverages are made from this varietal.

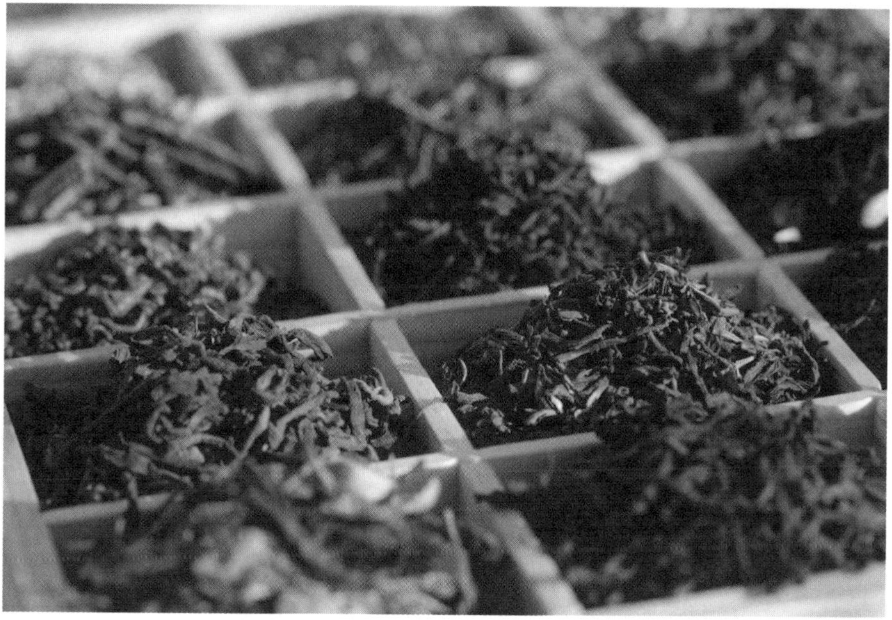

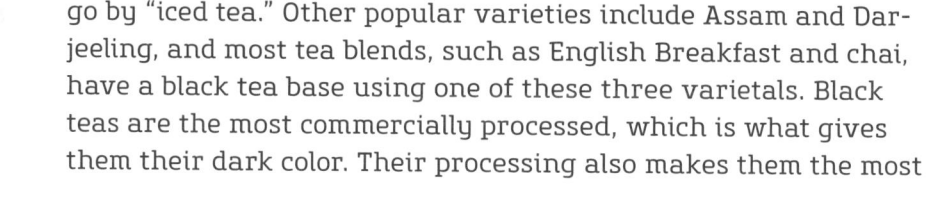

Ceylon is the type used for most commercially iced brews that just go by "iced tea." Other popular varieties include Assam and Darjeeling, and most tea blends, such as English Breakfast and chai, have a black tea base using one of these three varietals. Black teas are the most commercially processed, which is what gives them their dark color. Their processing also makes them the most

shelf stable of the teas, staying flavorful for several years in your cupboard.

GREEN: Known for its L-theanine content, green tea is a somewhat relaxed tea because of just that. L-theanine is an amino acid that creates calm in the brain while also stimulating your ability to think clearly. Amazing, huh? Green tea has been studied extensively in recent years, and it has been found beneficial for treating ailments such as obesity and diabetes. Popular types of green tea include sencha and hojicha as well as a tea-rice blend called genmaicha.

MATCHA: If it's just green tea, why am I giving matcha its own heading? Yes, matcha is a type of green tea, but there is one major difference that sets it apart from its colleagues: where with other teas you steep the leaves and then strain them, matcha is sold as a powder and you ingest the entire plant. What this boils down to (pun intended!) is more caffeine and more antioxidants, because, well, you're getting so much more of the plant. Because it is sold as a powder, matcha lends itself particularly well to cooking and baking.

WHITE: White tea is the most minimally processed form of tea. It is made from young tea leaves whose buds haven't fully opened, and those buds are covered in tiny hairs that, you guessed it, are

white. Because this tea is not allowed to darken and age, meaning it hasn't oxidized before being heated and dried, it yields a lighter color than other teas when brewed. White tea is steeped for less time, has a more delicate flavor, and is a pretty yellow or light green in the cup.

DOES HERBAL COUNT AS TEA?

Though they are called teas, herbal teas are not, by definition, really tea. The name *tisane* is used to denote leaves from plants other than *Camellia Sinensis* that are brewed and steeped in the fashion of tea. Hibiscus tea, for example, is made of flowers; rooibos is a shrub in the pea family; and holy basil, while sometimes available mixed with tea, is a green plant similar to culinary basil. While herbal tisanes have their own benefits, they don't have that essential wake-up component, caffeine. That's why the recipes in this chapter stick to real tea.

RECIPES

ORANGEY GREY TEA POPS

You may or may not have grown up with orange juice frozen into popsicle molds as a standard summer treat, which you thought were totally normal orange popsicles until going to a friend's house and seeing neon-bright plastic tubes of sweetness in their freezer. That's my story anyway, and I have to say, of all the "health foodie" snacks I grew up with, an O.J. pop was one that I was always eager to get my hands on.

This somewhat more adult version combines everyone's favorite breakfast juice with Earl Grey tea. These flavors pair perfectly because this type of tea is flavored with bergamot, a bitter orange citrus fruit that's grown in Europe. Bergamot is great for digestion, and studies have shown that it's also antimicrobial, anti-inflammatory, pain relieving, and heart healthy. This is, of course, in addition to the other antioxidant properties of the black tea that serves as Earl Grey's base, and the blood-pressure-reducing, immune-improving benefits of orange juice. Who knew a little popsicle could be so full of big health bennies?!

MAKES 8 STANDARD-SIZE POPSICLES

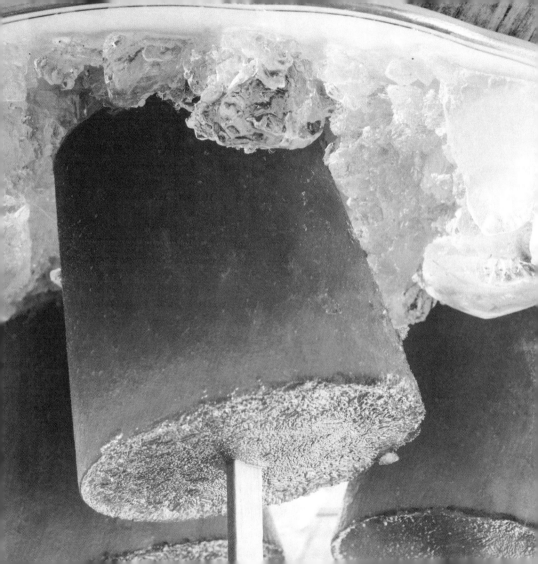

INGREDIENTS

2 tea bags Earl Grey or other black tea

½ cup (120 ml) nearly boiling water

¾ cup (180 ml) orange juice

1 cup (240 ml) cold water

INSTRUCTIONS

1. Brew the tea bags in the hot water for 3 to 4 minutes, then remove and discard the tea bags. Let cool.

2. In a mixing bowl, combine the orange juice with the brewed tea and cold water, stirring well.

3. Pour into popsicle molds and freeze until firm.

MATCHA CUPCAKES

On the one hand, these gluten- and grain-free paleo-ish cupcakes are shockingly healthy and yummy. On the other, there is over three-quarters of a serving (1 teaspoon) of matcha in every cupcake . . . so unlike some of the other treats in this book that are lovely lil' afternoon pick-me-ups, these cupcakes pack a fully caffeinated punch. While you can use culinary-grade matcha, I can't get over the gorgeous brightness of the ceremonial variety and find the swap worthwhile.

These cupcakes have an amazingly fluffy crumb, and I can attest to the fact that they stay fresh in the fridge for a solid week or more if your rationing abilities are similar to mine. The optional avocado frosting is for those who like their lilies gilded; I'm team "no frosting" when it comes to most sweets, but if you prefer cream atop your cake, you'll love this healthful topper.

MAKES 9 CUPCAKES

INGREDIENTS

DRY

1¼ cups (145 g) almond flour

¼ cup (30 g) coconut flour

2 tablespoons cane sugar

½ cup (100 g) Swerve or cane sugar, or a combo

2½ tablespoons matcha

1 teaspoon baking soda

½ teaspoon salt

WET

½ cup (120 ml) Greek yogurt (dairy or coconut)

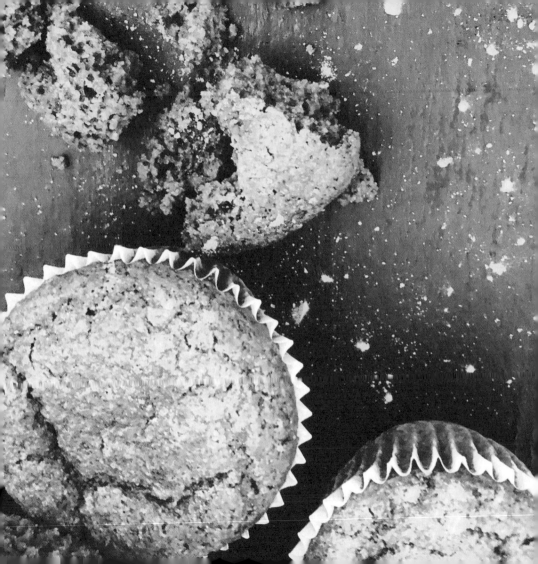

2 large eggs or vegan egg replacer equivalent

½ cup (120 ml) neutral oil, such as avocado or grape seed

1 teaspoon vanilla extract

⅓ cup almond milk

1 tablespoon cider vinegar

INSTRUCTIONS

1. Preheat the oven to 350°F (175°C).

2. In a large mixing bowl, combine all the dry ingredients with a fork or whisk, making sure no lumps of almond or coconut flour remain.

3. Add all the wet ingredients except the vinegar and stir until uniform in texture. Add the vinegar and stir well.

4. Pour the batter into nine wells of a cupcake pan (either with liners or greased), filling nearly all the way, and bake 25 to 30 minutes, or until an inserted knife comes out clean. If you are frosting (see below), let cool in pan before doing so.

OPTIONAL FROSTING INGREDIENTS

½ cup (75 g) avocado flesh

⅓ cup (75 ml) coconut oil

½ teaspoon matcha

¼ cup (50 g) Swerve or cane sugar

2 tablespoons almond milk

Small pinch salt

INSTRUCTIONS

In a blender, combine all the ingredients until smooth.

MATCHA-MINT GUMMIES

Have I stopped eating these gummies for even a single day since first testing them? Nope, nope, I haven't. They have been amalgamated right into my daily snack sitch, and I don't think they're going anywhere for a while.

While I'm a fan of canned goods generally never, I have to admit that when it comes to coconut milk, there's no comparison. In order to get the full-fat richness coconut milk can offer, it's got to come from a can, unless you make it yourself.

These gummies also contain a lot of gelatin, which is a form of collagen with lots of protein and amino acids. It has even proven successful for treating joint pain. Gelatin is also great for your hair and skin, as well as your brain. Since matcha is excellent for improving memory, this treat serves as tasty fuel for your mind and memory. Peppermint is stomach-soothing, invigorating, and gives these gummies a less grassy flavor than other matcha goods. Similar to the kombucha gelly candies, choose any mold you'd like, and remember that silicone is easiest for removal (or glass if using a pan).

MAKES 12 SERVINGS

INGREDIENTS

3 tablespoons plus 1½ teaspoons matcha

½ cup (75 g) powdered gelatin

3⅓ cups (795 ml) coconut milk, divided

1 teaspoon peppermint extract

Stevia or cane sugar to taste

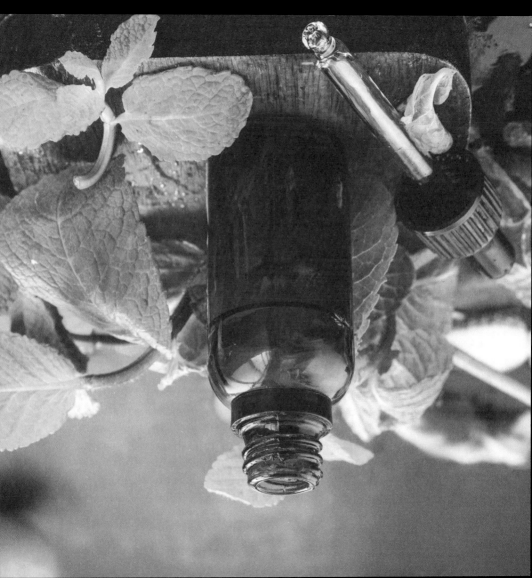

INSTRUCTIONS

1. Dissolve the matcha in 3 tablespoons of water; set aside.

2. In a saucepan, pour the gelatin over 2 cups (480 ml) of the coconut milk and ¼ cup (60 ml) water; let bloom for at least 5 minutes.

3. Place the saucepan over medium-low heat and add the remaining coconut milk, peppermint extract, and sweetener; stir until smooth and glossy. (If using sugar, I'd suggest 2 tablepsoons; if using stevia, 4 to 6 servings.)

4. Remove from the heat and add the matcha water, whisking until incorpo-rated. If any lumps of gelatin remain, strain the mixture.

5. Pour into molds or a pan, then refrigerate until firm, 2 to 4 hours. If using a pan, cut into shapes with a knife or cookie cutters. Store, refrigerated, in a tightly sealed container.

IRISH BREAKFAST FIZZ

For those times when you want tea but it just doesn't sound exciting enough, sparkling water is here to jazz things up. Breakfast teas in general carry a stronger flavor than afternoon teas, since they are meant to be drunk with a meal rather than enjoyed solo or with delicate tea-time foods. This recipe could be used for any tea, but the Assam/Ceylon blend of Irish Breakfast tea, with its malty character and bold finish, is a favorite of mine here. If you've ever been a morning soda drinker, this is a solid way to migrate that habit into a healthier one! Choose sparkling mineral water, and you add (no surprise) beneficial minerals to the drink.

MAKES 1 SERVING

INGREDIENTS

1 tea bag Irish Breakfast or other black tea

½ cup (120 ml) nearly boiling water

6–8 drops liquid stevia or 1½ teaspoons honey

Sparkling water

Wedge of lemon or orange, optional

INSTRUCTIONS

1. Brew the tea in the water for 3 to 4 minutes, then discard the tea bag and add the sweetener. Let the tea cool completely.

2. Fill a glass with ice; pour the tea in, then fill the glass with sparkling water. If desired, squeeze in a lemon or orange wedge.

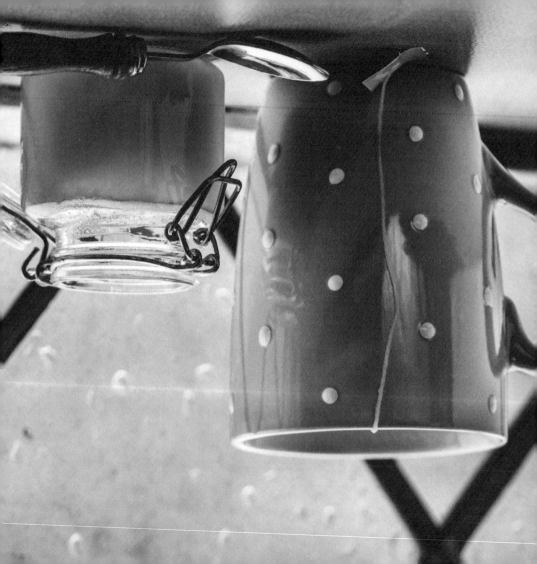

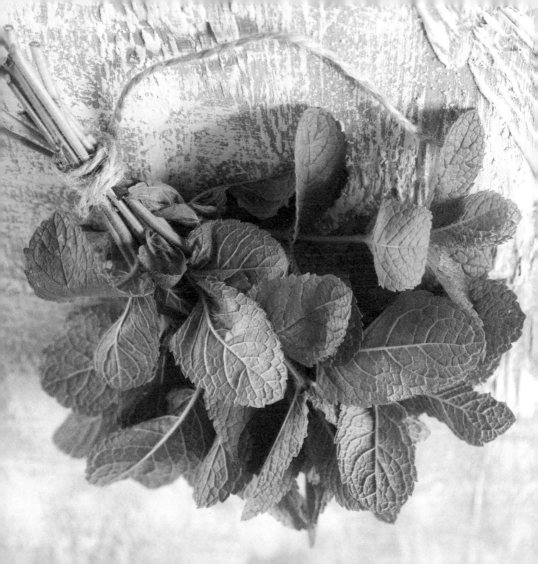

MOJITO ICED WHITE TEA

Ah, a refreshing mojito. Sounds good right about n—oh, wait, it's 9 a.m. For those of us who love mojito flavor but like to be conscious through the whole day, I present a nonalcoholic, iced tea version. White tea, with its mild flavor, is my choice here because it has very light caramel notes slightly similar to those of rum. Fresh mint is the main flavor of a mojito, and here you'll get all of its stomach-soothing and digestion-enhancing benefits without having those ruined by alcohol. Use liquid stevia for a vegan and sugarless version.

MAKES 1 SERVING

INGREDIENTS

1 tea bag white tea (I prefer jasmine)

½ cup (120 ml) nearly boiling water

1½ teaspoons honey

1 or more sprigs fresh mint

INSTRUCTIONS

1. Brew the tea in the water for 3 to 4 minutes, then discard the tea bag and add the honey. Let cool completely.

2. In a glass, muddle the mint sprig with ¼ cup (60 ml) of the brewed tea.

3. Leaving the mint spring in the glass, fill the glass with ice; add remaining tea concentrate, then enough water to fill. Stir well.

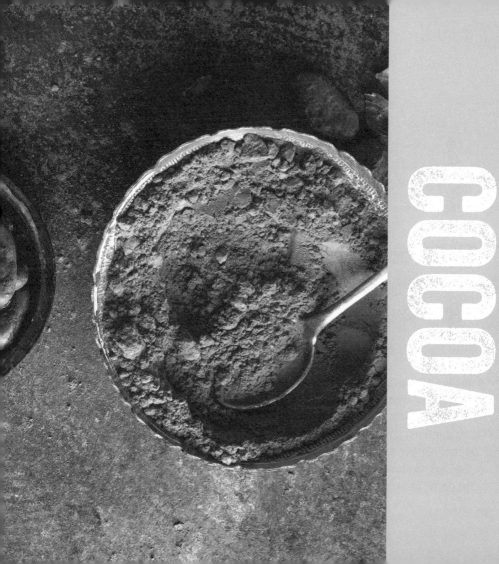

COCOA

CAFFEINE & MORE

On the one hand, yes, cocoa has caffeine, which makes cocoa-related foods such as chocolate great pick-me-ups. One tablespoon of cocoa powder, a.k.a. cocoa mass, has 12 milligrams of caffeine. That's not a ton, but the low caffeine content makes cocoa treats a safer option for later in the day, when you want something caffeinated but don't want the stress of possibly missing your bedtime.

On the other hand, in addition to caffeine, cocoa contains other elements that can make your day better, including:

THEOBROMINE: This stimulant is more concentrated in cocoa powder and dark chocolate than its milky counterparts. Theobromine can be found in other plants, too, such as tea, but it was discovered in chocolate in the 1800s and continues to be associated with that treat. The effects of theobromine are similar to those of caffeine, but theobromine stimulates your nervous system a little less than caffeine while acting more strongly on your heart. Theobromine is also thought to improve mood.

PHENETHYLAMINE: More commonly known as PEA, because seriously who wants to try and say that big long word, this compound creates the "love" high associated with chocolate. It stimulates the nervous system, releasing endorphins. It also increases dopamine activity, which is why it can simulate the "in love" feeling that chocolate is famous for.

ANANDAMIDE: Another word you probably don't want to have to say, anandamide is a cannabinoid found in only two places: chocolate and THC (the chemical in marijuana that makes you high, just in case you are really, really pure and didn't know that). Does the anandamide in chocolate have the ability to get you as high as smoking weed? Obviously not, or we'd all likely be a lot more accidentally stoned on the daily. You'd have to eat many pounds of chocolate to get the same effect as you do from smoking weed, but even in small doses, anandamide creates an uplifted, euphoric feeling.

Where Does Chocolate Come From?

Cocoa is a funny plant. We take the cacao bean, separate it into its varied products—cocoa butter and cocoa powder—then put those back together to create chocolate. While you can eat chocolate in its whole form before any of that happens, purchasable as either whole cacao beans or broken into cacao nibs, you probably don't

want to. They're about as tasty as 100 percent chocolate baking bars, which is to say they are chocolatey but not exactly delish, and their texture is pretty gritty.

Forms of Cacao

As mentioned above, chocolate is rarely used in its actual, whole form, or even in nibs, outside of the quirky world of raw food-ism. (Note that when I was eating raw, I ate those guys by the handful—they make you feel pretty kickass, plus when on a raw diet your conception of "yummy" changes significantly.) Because I wanted this to be accessible for the average Joe and cup of joe drinker, I've stuck to just the basic forms in this chapter, using just chocolate chips and cocoa powder.

Chocolate Chips: A Broad Category

Bittersweet, semisweet, baking, sugar free, dairy free, grain sweetened: there is no shortage of chocolate chip types out there! Without even getting into baking bars, your choices are mani-fold. Which should you use? These recipes are versatile and really, the best thing I can say is to choose based on your general tastes around chocolate. Like a darker bar or treat? Choose bittersweet, which has a higher cocoa content than semisweet. If you're more a

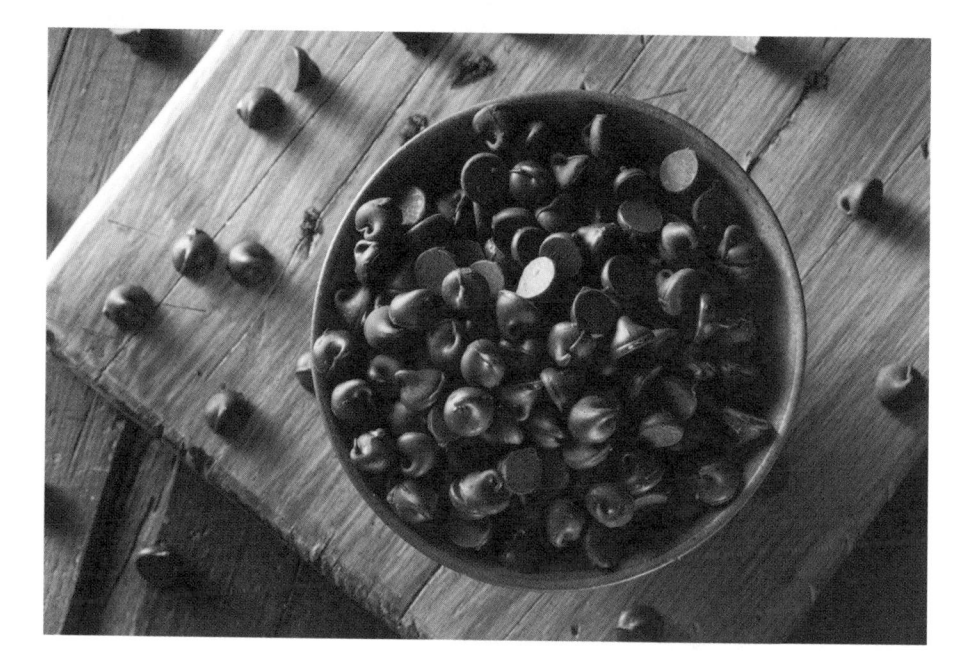

milk chocolate person, opt for semisweet, as it is sweeter because it is made with less cocoa mass. Going paleo? Get the stevia-sweetened ones, which I used in a 1:1 ratio with bittersweet when testing the recipes in this chapter. Typically you can sub out about half the quantity without your audience realizing you've tricked them, so I take the opportunity whenever possible. Grain sweet-

ened are the safest choice for vegans, since white sugar processing is often not vegan.

The Powdered Stuff

The two main types of cocoa powder are alkalized, a.k.a. "Dutch process," and non-alkalized, or "natural." In short, alkalized is a more processed, prettier product, and non-alkalized is better for you. The difference is exactly what it sounds like: alkalized is processed with alkali, which reduces its acidity while enhancing its dark color. Non-alkalized retains more of the stuff in cocoa that is good for you, as it is less processed. The darker the cocoa powder, the more harshly it was processed: black cocoa, which is used in things like Oreo cookies, is as dark as it gets.

The recipes in this chapter were tested with natural, non-alkalized cocoa powder, which is available just as widely as the other kind. I like that it has a stronger flavor and more health bennies; I consider the color amply dark. None of these recipes were tested with raw cacao powder, but if it's your preference, give it a shot!

CRUNCHY RICE BARK

Sometimes in life, you just need to lighten things up a bit. Chocolate is an intense food that can quickly overwhelm a recipe if you choose a darker variety, but the crispy brown rice cereal turns this bark from heavyweight to featherweight while adding fiber, zinc, and vitamin B. I chose dried apricots to add a sweet-and-sour chew factor in addition to more fiber and vitamin A. You could also use raisins, cranberries, or even dried cherries if you're feeling fancy.

MAKES ABOUT 16 PIECES BARK

INGREDIENTS

2 cups (350 g) chocolate chips

1 cup (15 g) rice cereal (I used crispy sprouted brown rice)

½ cup (65 g) diced dried apricots

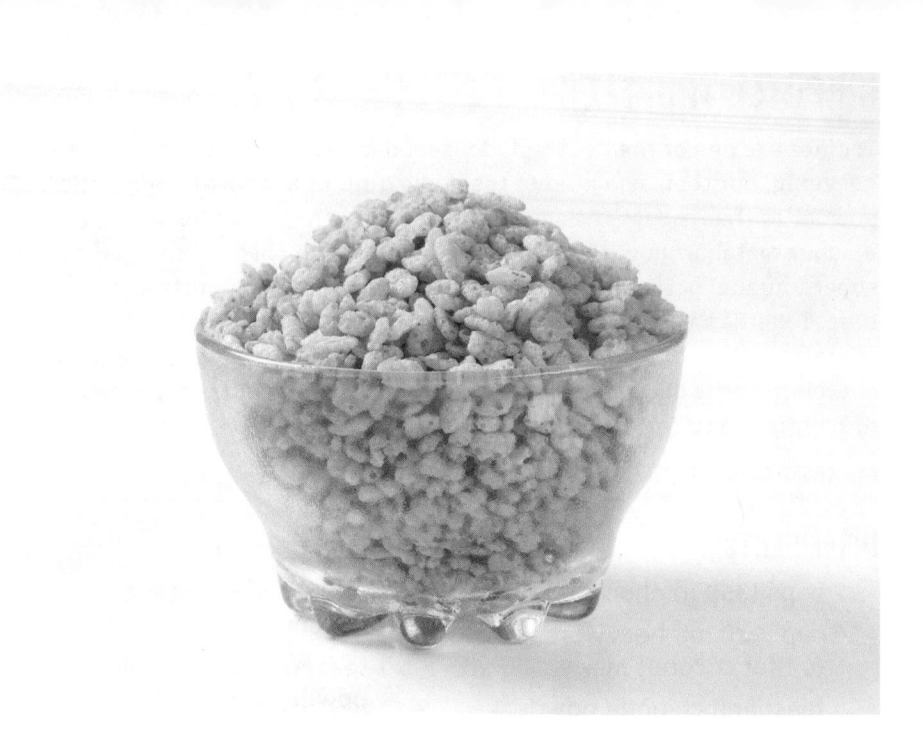

INSTRUCTIONS

1. In a saucepan over low heat or in the top of a double boiler over simmering water, melt the chocolate chips.

2. Remove from the heat and add the cereal and apricots.

3. Pour the mixture onto a lined baking sheet (any size works since it won't take up a whole pan) and refrigerate until firm, then break into pieces.

CHIPOTLE TRUFFLES

Truffles are one of the heaviest, densest dessert bites around. They're heavenly, but they also kind of taste like guilt in a mouthful. Chipotle powder to the rescue! The smoked jalapeño in these truffles will speed up your metabolism with its heat while offering a spice factor that tastes super unusual yet manages to pair perfectly with the uplifting cacao base. Together, they make for an invigorating truffle. I love chili and chocolate together so much that I almost always have a disc of Guajillo chocolate in the chocolate drawer of my fridge. (Yes, I have a chocolate drawer in my fridge, for reals.)

MAKES ABOUT 2 DOZEN TRUFFLES

INGREDIENTS

2 cups (350 g) chocolate chips

½ cup (120 ml) heavy cream or full-fat coconut milk

½ teaspoon chipotle powder, plus a pinch

1 tablespoon butter or coconut oil

1 teaspoon ancho chile powder, optional, for additional chile flavor

1 tablespoon cocoa powder

INSTRUCTIONS

1. In a saucepan over low heat, combine all the ingredients except the cocoa powder and pinch of chipotle powder, and melt until smooth.

2. Refrigerate until set, at least 1 hour.

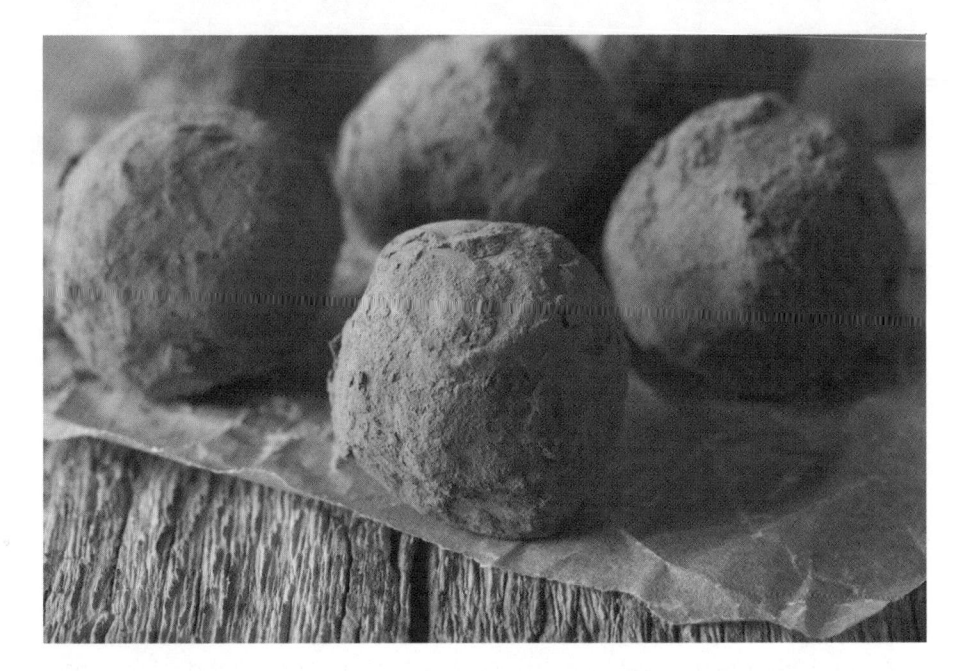

3. Combine the cocoa powder with the pinch of chipotle powder and spread on a small plate.

4. Using a melon baller or a spoon, scoop the chocolate. Roll gently into balls, then coat in the cocoa-chipotle mixture. Refrigerate in a sealed container until ready to eat.

CHOCOLATE STOUT CHILI

No meat is no problem when you want a chili that reads as a hardy indulgence but doesn't involve any animal products. This chili gets its deep, dark flavor from a double hit of chocolate by way of cocoa powder and chocolate stout. (The cocoa is more important than the beer, so if you only have access to a plain stout like Guinness, don't stress.) Beans give their fiber and protein, chilies both fresh and dried power up your metabolism, and cocoa adds a little lift so the dish doesn't give you any of the sleepy feels that chili otherwise can. The alcohol in the beer cooks mostly out, so don't worry about getting the wrong kind of buzz!

MAKES 4 LARGE OR 6 SMALL SERVINGS

INGREDIENTS

- 1 tablespoon neutral oil, such as avocado or grape seed
- ½ cup (65 g) diced onion
- ½ cup (75 g) diced bell pepper
- 1 tablespoon minced garlic
- 1 cup (177 g) cooked kidney beans
- 1 cup (171 g) cooked pinto beans
- 1 cup (240 ml) chocolate stout beer

- 1 cup (240 ml) jarred tomato puree
- 2 tablespoons tomato paste
- 2–4 tablespoons diced jalapeños or serranos (quantity to taste)
- 2 tablespoons chili powder
- 2 tablespoons cocoa powder
- 1 teaspoon smoked paprika
- 1 teaspoon salt
- ¼ teaspoon chipotle powder, optional

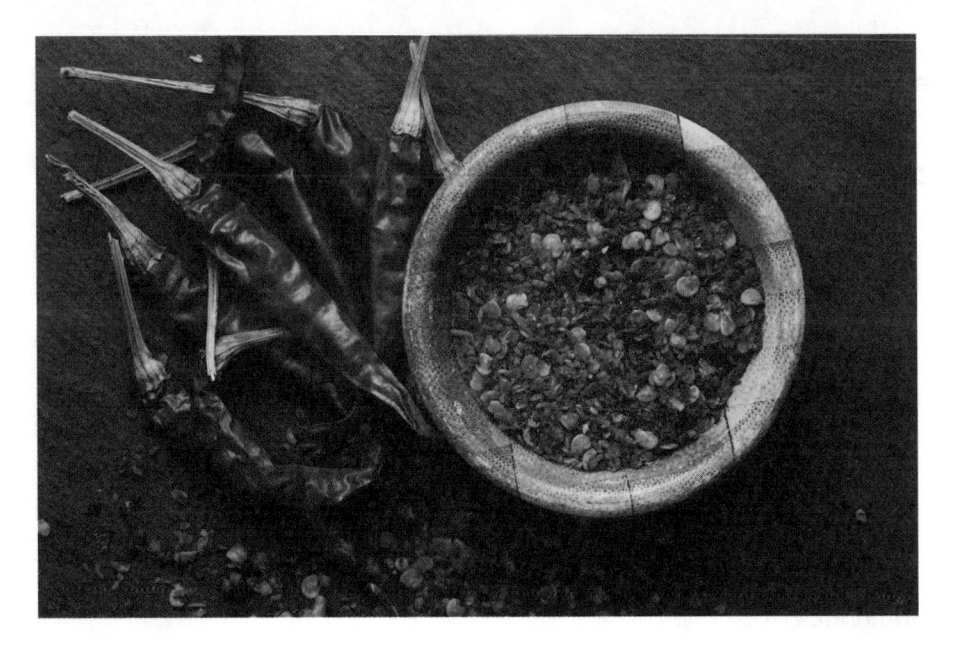

INSTRUCTIONS

1. In a medium pot, heat the oil over medium-high heat.

2. Add the onion and saute for 5 minutes, until softened.

3. Add the bell pepper and garlic and saute for 1 minute.

4. Add the remaining ingredients, stir well, and bring to a boil.

5. Reduce the heat to a simmer and cook 15 minutes more, stirring occasionally, until the chili has darkened.

BREAKFAST BROWNIES

Confession: I have zero interest in breakfast. I'm an intermittent faster who pours a world's supply of whipping cream in her coffee, or does Bulletproof (see page 34), and begins contemplating food around noon. However, I love breakfast foods. Waffles, pancakes, chilaquiles? Give them all to me . . . at dinner time. So I'm here to say that while these brownies are healthy and filling enough for breakfast, they totally work at any time of day. This is one of those "fool everyone" recipes, where no one will believe that there's no flour or added oil. Beyond being chocolatey to the nth degree, they're high in protein, moderate in carbs and fat, and full of nutrition thanks to sweet potatoes, oats, protein powder, nut butter, and eggs or a vegan egg replacer equivalent. If you're looking for a frosted version, try topping them with the chocolate hummus recipe (page 89).

MAKES 12 LARGE BROWNIES

INGREDIENTS

- 1 cup (240 ml) mashed, cooked sweet potato
- 2 eggs or vegan egg replacer equivalent
- ½ cup (120 ml) nut butter, crunchy or smooth
- ½ cup (50 g) protein powder
- ⅓ cup (30 g) cocoa powder
- ½ teaspoon baking soda
- ½ teaspoon salt
- ½ teaspoon vanilla extract
- ¾ cup (65 g) rolled oats
- ½ cup (85 g) chocolate chips, optional

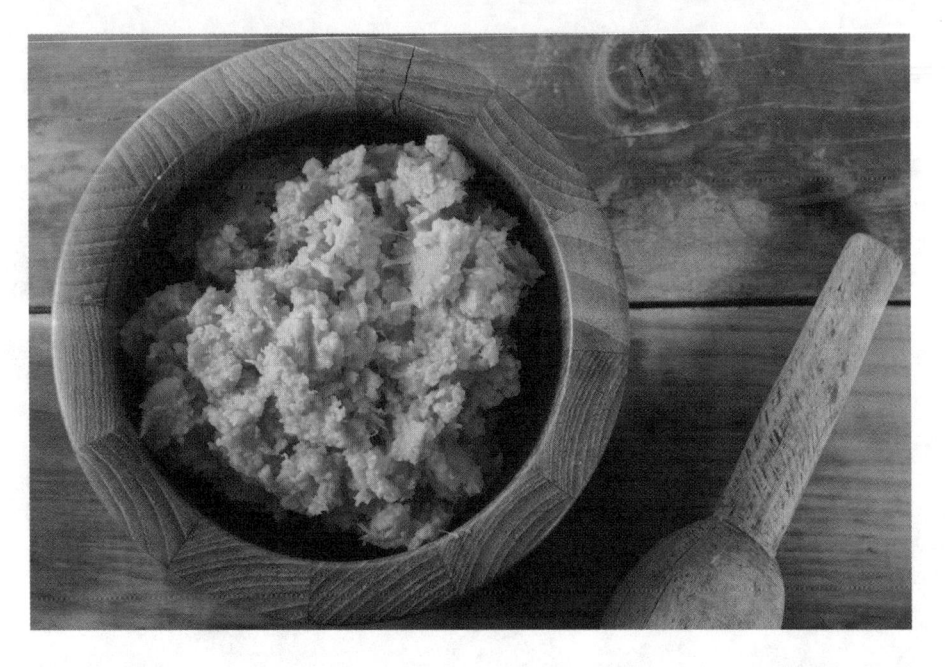

INSTRUCTIONS

1. Preheat the oven to 325°F (165°C).

2. Place all the ingredients except the oats and optional chocolate chips in a food processor or blender and process or blend until uniform in texture.

3. Stir in the oats and chocolate chips, if using, until incorporated.

4. Pour the batter into a greased 8-inch (20 cm) square baking dish and bake about 40 minutes, or until an inserted knife comes out clean.

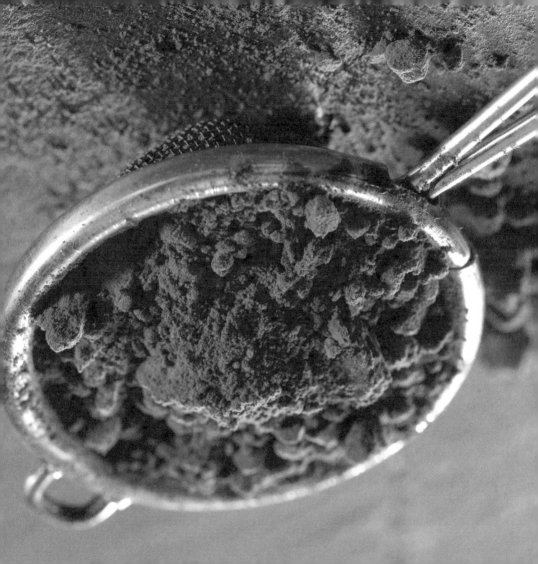

CHOCOLATE HUMMUS

I have to admit that when the dessert hummus trend hit, I was not the first person to board the train to creamy, sweet bean town. Even though I've been making chickpea and black bean chocolate cakes since the 1990s (that random skill is how I got my first chef job at age 19), the idea of an uncooked version didn't fly with me initially. This recipe took some work—and rework—to get me to a place where I was comfortable endorsing dessert bean spread. But after deciding to use black beans over chickpeas for color and smoothness as well as for their anthocyanins (the antioxidants in purple-black foods that give them their color), I got my ticket for the dessert hummus train. Then, when I added maple syrup to sweeten the deal while adding some minerals and cinnamon to keep that syrup from hitting your blood sugar levels too hard, I was all aboard.

MAKES 8 SERVINGS

INGREDIENTS

2 cups (370 g) cooked black beans

¼ cup plus 1 tablespoon (75 g) almond or other milk

¼ cup (25 g) cocoa powder

¼ cup (60 ml) maple syrup

½ teaspoon cinnamon

Large pinch salt

INSTRUCTIONS

In a food processor or blender, combine all the ingredients until uniform in texture.

CHOCOLATE PROTEIN MILK

Chocolate milk is a nostalgic drink that doesn't have much to offer health-wise beyond some protein and fortified vitamins. But you can turn that dessert-y snack into something functional while getting a nice little theobromine boost with this chocolate protein milk. It's perfect for when you want a protein drink but don't necessarily feel like having a thick smoothie. If your protein powder dissolves easily, this can be made in a mason jar with a lid, which means you don't have to dirty any extra dishes. Swap out chocolate protein for a berry one, and you'll get a mixed flavor reminiscent of Neapolitan ice cream.

MAKES 1 SERVING

INGREDIENTS

1 cup (240 ml) milk (dairy or non)

1 scoop chocolate protein powder

1½ tablespoons cocoa powder

Stevia or maple syrup to taste, if desired

INSTRUCTIONS

In a shaker cup or blender, combine all the ingredients until smooth.

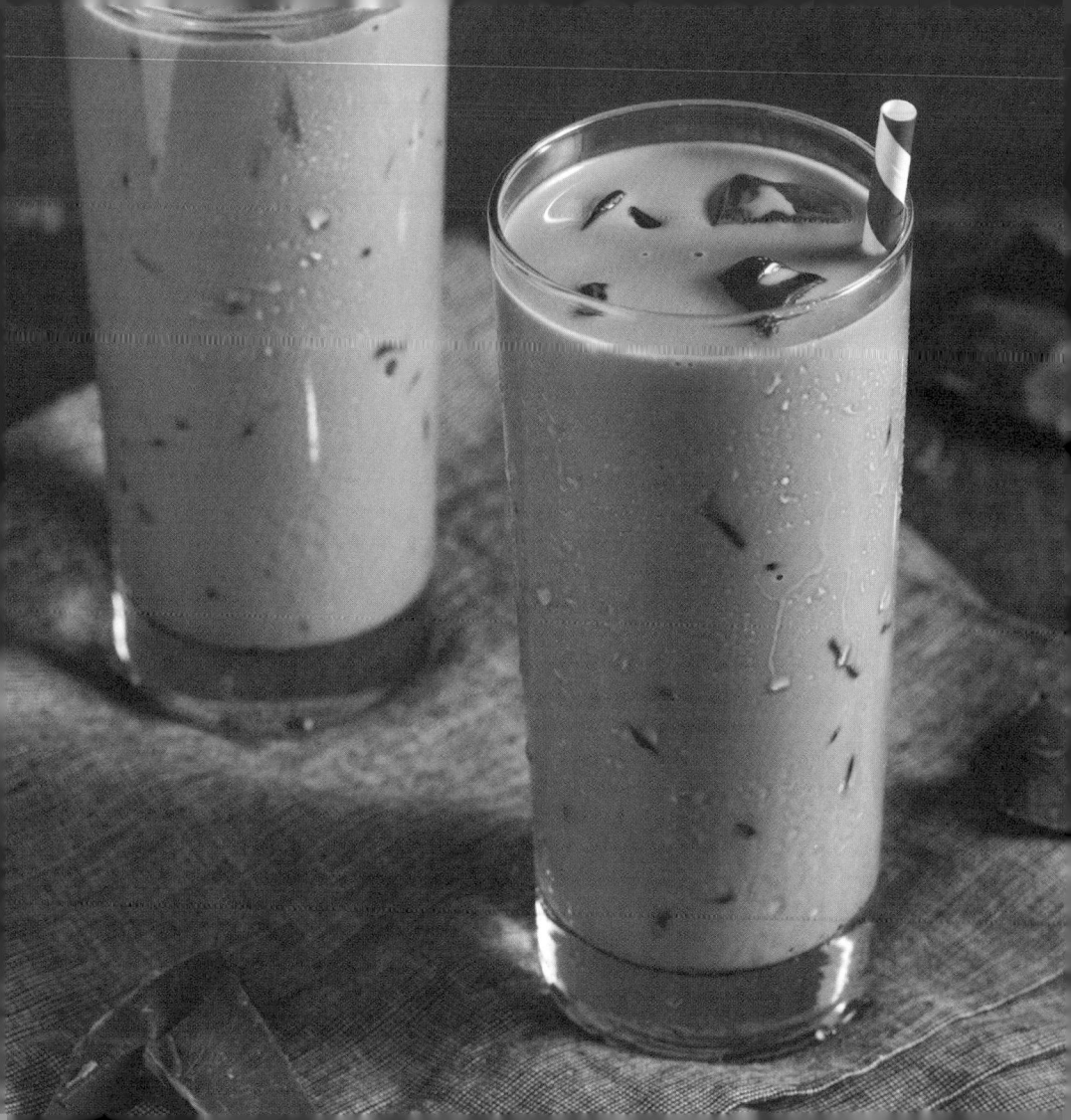

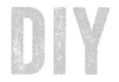

DIY

WHAT'S THE BIG DIY-EAL?

If you're at all crafty or have even just visited sites like Pinterest that highlight homemade goods, you definitely know that there are countless recipes for homemade bath and beauty products. While commercial brands will charge by the ounce, or even by the fraction of the ounce, you can often make your own by the pound for far less than an ounce of a single-purchase product. Sure, there are some commercial products worth buying, but the products in this chapter are all so easy to make that you might as well try them out as quick replacements for things you would otherwise have to purchase.

JUST BREATHE

Scents have extremely evocative powers. They can be agents of nostalgia, calling up memories that go all the way back to child-hood. The neurological responses we have to different smells are

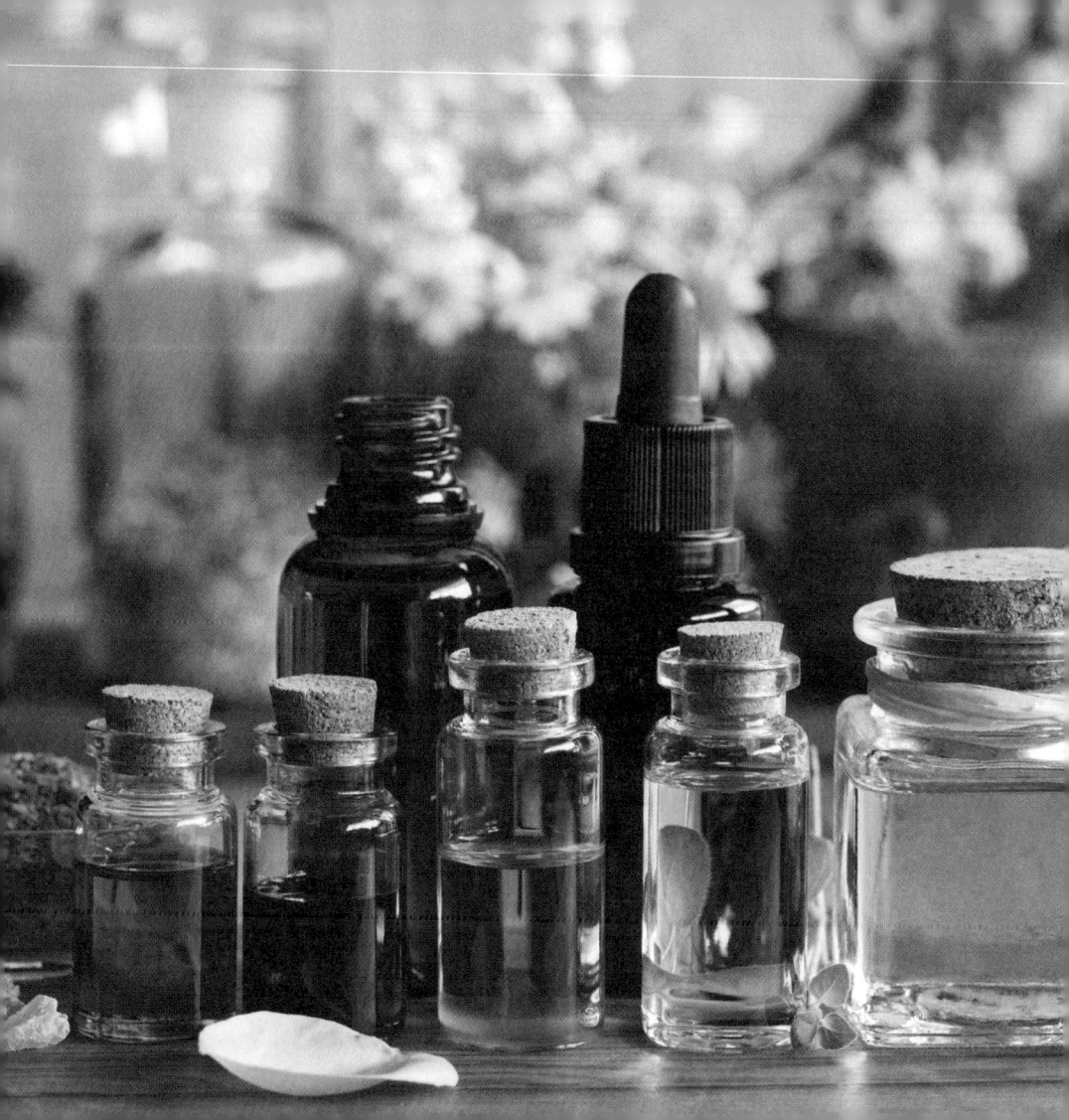

definitely intense, and it has been shown that a smell will trigger stronger emotions and more vivid recollections of an event than an image will. Our sense of smell is also more acute and more sensitive than any of our other senses, so it isn't too big of a surprise that using scents can give us jolts of energy, clearing the fog and bringing a sleepy mind back to full wakefulness.

OIL FOR EASE

There are plenty of ways to get a scent into your DIY bath and beauty products, but the purest and simplest one is to use essential oils. Essential oils are concentrated versions of plants that have been boiled down . . . and down . . . and down until just a drop or two is enough to have a potent impact. Some oils incite a relaxed response in our bodies and brains, which you'll learn about on the *Sleep* side. Others have a wake-up effect, and those are the ones used in this chapter.

When it comes to picking oils, I prefer organic and non-GMO versions, because you're putting them on your body, and it's always best to not breathe in or slather on something full of concentrated pesticides. There are many reputable brands, but for some reason, the best ones are multi-level-marketing based and have to be ordered through a human rather than a website or

store. My advice here is to generally avoid inexpensive internet-based brands, or generic ones you find at bath and body care shops. In my experience, they just don't smell as good and tend to be cut with other oils. Do your research. It'll be worth it!

WAKE-UP ESSENCES

I didn't want to go hog wild suggesting you buy more than a couple of oils for any given recipe in this chapter, so I kept the projects pretty minimal, with just one or two oils each. However, there are scads of essential oils that are great for brightening up your day and energizing you! Essential oils that have qualities to help you perk up, some of which are used in this chapter, include: citrus, mint, rosemary, basil, ginger, cinnamon, juniper, thyme, eucalyptus, black pepper, and pine. Feel free to swap out any of the ones I suggest for oils you prefer the aroma of, though of course exercise caution. When they say "volatile" compounds on the label, they aren't joking! Never put anything with inherent heat, such as black pepper oil or cinnamon, on your skin unless heavily diluted.

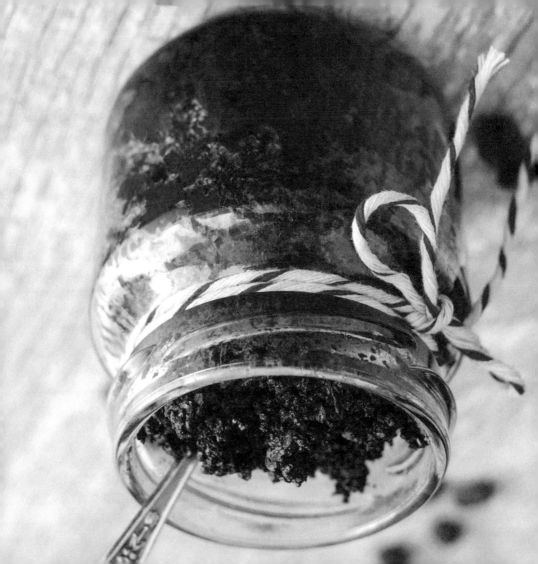

DIY RECIPES

COFFEE BODY SCRUB

Body scrubs have taken off in recent years, and I'm of the opinion that there's no reason at all to buy something for $20 (or more) that you can make in less than 5 minutes for less than a dollar. The added bonuses of DIYing are that you can scent it as you wish, and you can control the ingredients—have you ever thought about the GMO factor in relation to the sugar or oil you rub on your body? Now you don't have to!

The equal parts coffee, sugar, and oil in this recipe will give you an invigorating shower experience that sets your day off to a feisty start. And while this scrub won't clear any cellulite forever, it does a surprisingly good job of temporarily reducing it thanks to coffee's caffeine content.

MAKES APPROXIMATELY 1 CUP (190 G) SCRUB

INGREDIENTS

⅓ cup (30 g) ground coffee

⅓ cup (75 g) brown sugar

⅓ cup (75 ml) neutral oil, such as avocado or grape seed

1 teaspoon honey

10 drops essential oil: mint, citrus, or wood

INSTRUCTIONS

Mix all the ingredients together in a mixing bowl, then store in an airtight container.

FRESH FACE TONER

I'm a big fan of DIY face products, but most tend to have a very short shelf life. Vitamin C, for example, oxidizes within a week or two in the cabinet, and the effort of walking to the fridge every time I wash my face is not one I'm able to commit to. That's why I came up with this enlivening toner that is made from shelf-stable ingredients that will easily keep until you use it up.

A spray bottle makes life feel like a spa; just spritz a bit onto your face in the morning after a shower or washing your face. The witch hazel reduces inflammation and oil, the aloe vera soothes skin and relieves redness, and the citrus oils combat the bacteria that cause acne while simultaneously brightening your skin and uplifting your mood. Distilled water is ideal, but spring water will do, too—just avoid tap.

MAKES 2 OUNCES (60 ML) SPRAY

INGREDIENTS

2 tablespoons witch hazel

½ teaspoon aloe vera gel

20–25 drops citrus essential oil (grapefruit, lemon, orange, or a combo)

INSTRUCTIONS

Pour all the ingredients plus 2 tablespoons water into a 2-ounce (60 ml) spray bottle and shake well; shake before each use.

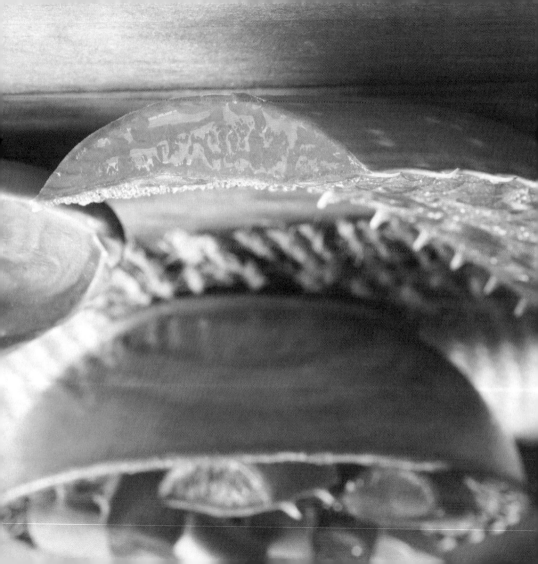

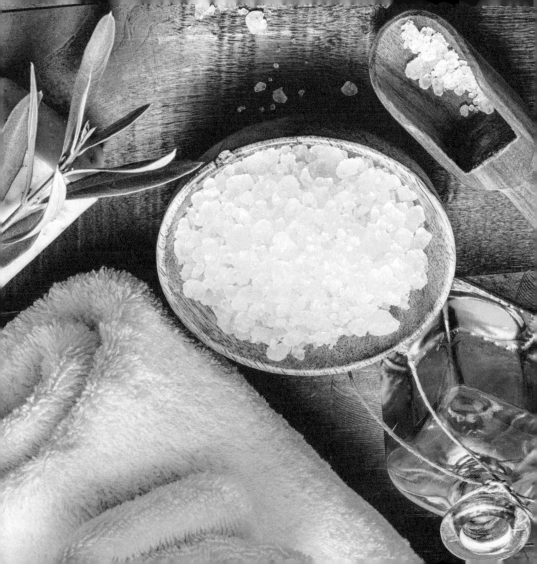

ENERGIZING BATH SALTS

Without anything added for fragrance, bath salts are just, well, salts and some baking soda. When you purchase bath salts, a big part of the appeal is how good they smell. (If by some chance you're a person who dislikes fragrance, this is an awesome opportunity for you, because you can make yours unscented!) Even though a morning bath isn't the most common thing in the world, what if it could be? What if on a self-care Saturday or Sunday Funday, you had the option of lounging in a tub filled with bath salts that would perk you up instead of wind you down? Sounds kind of fun, no? I certainly thought so, so I created this energizing bath salt blend that will take you about half a minute to make. This amount is perfect for one soak, but if you want salts on demand, you can double or triple the ingredients proportionally, as this recipe will keep for a long time when tightly sealed in a jar.

MAKES ABOUT 1¼ CUPS (300 G) BATH SALTS

INGREDIENTS

1 cup (240 g) epsom salts

¼ cup (60 g) sea salt

1 tablespoon baking soda

10 drops bergamot or other citrus essential oil

1–2 drops wintergreen or other mint essential oil

INSTRUCTIONS

Mix all the ingredients together in a bowl, then store in an airtight container until use.

EUCALYPTUS SHOWER SPRAY

Eucalyptus is known for helping clear your sinuses when you have a cold, but that's not all it's good for! This oil opens your lungs, helping you get more air into them, which will definitely wake you up. It also kills mold and bacteria, meaning the steam in your shower will further cleanse you (and your tiles). Vodka is used not to get you a little buzzed (you won't feel its effects at all, I promise) but to emulsify the oil into the water. That said, you'll still want to shake it before each use. As with the toner spray, choose distilled or spring water, not tap. While the recipe seems like a small quantity, you only need a few spritzes once your shower water is hot, so it will last for many a morning.

MAKES 1 OUNCE (30 ML) SPRAY

INGREDIENTS

1 tablespoon vodka

1 tablespoon water

10 drops eucalyptus oil

INSTRUCTIONS

Pour all the ingredients into a 1-ounce (30 ml) bottle and shake well; shake before each use.

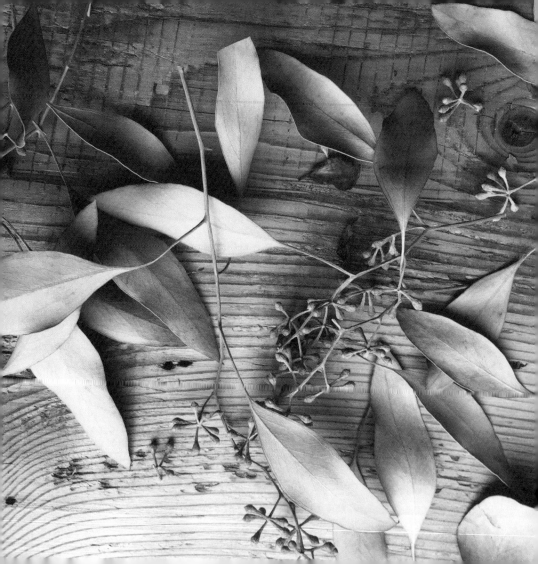

ACKNOWLEDGMENTS

A friend told me recently that, because I'm an unusually complex human, I am "a village trapped in the body of a woman." While I love the poetry of that—and did, in fact, use that line in a poem I wrote a week later—I must acknowledge that I've been assisted by many helpful additional villagers who have made this book's journey possible, including but not limited to:

COLEEN O'SHEA, MY LITERARY AGENT: Thank you for your continued, unwavering faith in me, and for your ability to help publishers believe that no, really, I can write entire books in about a month, and it'll go super well.

ANN TREISTMAN, MY EDITOR AT COUNTRYMAN PRESS: Thank you for having enough interest in working with me to suss out what the right projects would be, and for being so fastidious and awesome to work with for all my inquiries throughout the process.

ELISETTE CARLSON/SMACK! MEDIA: Eli, I can't count the ways you've been instrumental in my career, and I'll keep doing my best to make it worth your while.

ALECIA/P!NK: Working with you changed me so much, and all for the better. Most relevant to this book, thank you for the mind space that working with you put me in, and for cosmically making the timing of when I needed to write this line up so perfectly with when you left for your tour.

MY FAMILY: You are where my purpose was found, and your pride fuels me.

MANDY: My bestie, my sous chef, my food soulmate, I love you so much and am so happy you could be part of this project. Thank you for all your help, and I can't wait to do it again!

SAT DEVBIR SINGH: My magical starseed sibling, your healing work continues to facilitate all the good stuff in my life.

ZOFIA: You are my longest-ever working relationship by several years now! Thank you for showing me that I can commit to something long term—as long as no one ever mentions that that's what's happening—and for the matcha gummies idea.

ALEX: Thank you for the lashings, verbal and otherwise, to keep my butt in gear on this, for offering up the role of being my go-to without batting an eye, and for having all it took to be the main muse of a girl whose attention was otherwise impossible to keep.

MY PEOPLE: There's a good bunch of you between SF and LA and NYC, and I know you'll see this; you always buy my books because you are wonderful friends. Thank you for your unwavering presence in my life.

MY BABIES: Chanty and Bechamel, without you I'd just be a crazy cat-less lady. Who else could have given me such good company for the last month as I barely left the house writing this?

YOU: My sincere appreciation to everyone who picked up this book. You are why I'm here, why I do what I do. Without you, there would be no one for me to help feel better, and that would be no life for me. Thank you so much for wanting to hear what I have to say; I hope it contributes to your wellness and happiness.

REFERENCES

Introduction (Wake)

Africa House. "The History of Coffee." https://www.africaresource.com/house/index.php/news/our-announcements/21-the-history-of-coffee.

Kalda, A., L. Yu, E. Oztas, and J. F. Chen. "Novel Neuroprotection by Caffeine and Adenosine A(2A) Receptor Antagonists in Animal Models of Parkinson's Disease." *Journal of Neurological Science*, no. 248 (Oct. 2006): 9–15.

Kuakini Health System. "Caffeine: America's Most Popular Drug." https://www.kuakini.org/wps/portal/public/Health-Wellness/Health-Info-Tips/Miscellaneous/Caffeine--America-s-Most-Popular-Drug.

Mitchell, D. C., C. A. Knight, J. Hockenberry, R. Teplansky, and T. J. Hartman. "Beverage Caffeine Intakes in the U.S." *Food and Chemical Toxicology*, no. 63 (January 2014): 136–142.

Ruxton, C. H. S. "The Impact of Caffeine On Mood, Cognitive Function, Performance and Hydration: A Review of Benefits and Risks." *Nutrition Bulletin*, no. 33 (March 2008): 15–25.

UK Tea & Infusions Association. "The Birth of Tea in China." http://www.tea.co.uk/tea-a-brief-history#china.

Vail, Gabrielle. "The Food of the Gods: Cacao Use among the Prehispanic Maya." Mexicolore (website). http://www.mexicolore.co.uk/maya/chocolate/cacao-use-among-the-prehispanic-maya.

Wilcox, A. R. "The Effects of Caffeine and Exercise on Body Weight, Fat-Pad Weight, and Fat-Cell Size." *Medicine and Science in Sports and Exercise*, no. 14 (1982): 317–21.

Xu, Kui, Yue-Hang Xu, Jiang-Fan Chen, and Michael A. Schwarzschild. "Neuroprotection by Caffeine: Time Course and Role of Its Metabolites in the MPTP Model of Parkinson's Disease." *Neuroscience*, no. 167 (May 2010): 475–81.

Coffee

Eskelinen, M. H., and M. Kivipelto. "Caffeine as a Protective Factor in Dementia and Alzheimer's Disease." *Journal of Alzheimer's Disease*, no. 20 (2010; Suppl. 1): S167–74.

Gapstur, S. M., et al. "Associations of Coffee Drinking and Cancer Mortality in the Cancer Prevention Study-II." *Cancer Epidemiology Biomarkers & Prevention*, 26 (2017): 10.1158/1055-9965.EPI=17=0353.

Gunter, Marc J., et al. "Coffee Drinking and Mortality in 10 European Countries: A Multinational Cohort Study." *Annals of Internal Medicine*, no. 167 (2017): 236–47.

Heng-Quan, Ran, Jun-Zhou Wang, and Chang-Qin Sun. "Coffee Consumption and Pancreatic Cancer Risk: An Update Meta-analysis of Cohort Studies." *Pakistan Journal of Medical Sciences*, no. 32 (Jan.–Feb. 2016): 253–9.

Xie, F., D. Wang, Z. Huang, and Y. Guo. "Coffee Consumption and Risk of Gastric Cancer: A Large Updated Meta-Analysis of Prospective Studies." *Nutrients*, no. 18 (Sep. 2014): 3734–46.

Introduction (Sleep)

Bazar, K. A., A. J. Yun, and P. Y. Lee. "Debunking a Myth: Neurohormonal and Vagal Modulation of Sleep Centers, Not Redistribution of Blood Flow, May Account for Postprandial Somnolence." *Medical Hypotheses*, no. 63 (2004): 778–82.

Roth, Thomas. "Insomnia: Definition, Prevalence, Etiology, and Consequences." *Journal of Clinical Sleep Medicine*, no. 3 (Aug. 2007; Suppl. 5): S7–10.

Nibble

Geddes, Linda. "Why We Need a Siesta After Dinner." *New Scientist* (online), June 5, 2006. https://www.newscientist.com/article/dn9272-why-we-need-a-siesta-after-dinner.

Hansen, Anita L., et al. "Fish Consumption, Sleep, Daily Functioning, and Heart Rate Variability." *Journal of Clinical Sleep Medicine*, no. 10 (May 2014): 567–75.

Littleton, Philip. "Unveiling a Thanksgiving Fallacy." SiOWfa15 (blog), November 29, 2015. https://sites.psu.edu/siowfa15/2015/11/29/unveiling-a-thanksgiving-fallacy.

Schmidt, J. A., et al. "Plasma Concentrations and Intakes of Amino Acids in Male Meat-Eaters, Fish-Eaters, Vegetarians and Vegans: A Cross-Sectional Analysis in the EPIC-Oxford Cohort." *European Journal of Clinical Nutrition*, no. 70, (2016): 306–12.

Xiao, Fei, et al. "Effects of Essential Amino Acids on Lipid Metabolism in Mice and

Humans." *Journal of Molecular Endocrinology*, no. 57 (Nov. 2016): 223–31. http://jme.endocrinology-journals.org/content/57/4/223.full.

Spoon

Hou, Yongqing, Yulong Yin, and Guoyao Wu. "Dietary Essentiality of 'Nutritionally Non-Essential Amino Acids' for Animals and Humans." *Experimental Biology and Medicine*, 240 (Aug. 2015): 997–1007.

Trivedi, M. S., et al. "Food-Derived Opioid Peptides Inhibit Cysteine Uptake with Redox and Epigenetic Consequences." *The Journal of Nutritional Biochemistry*, no. 25, issue 10 (October 2014): 1011–18.

Sip

American Academy of Sleep Science. "Study Suggests That What You Eat Can Influence How You Sleep." Press release, January 14, 2016. https://aasm.org/study-suggests-that-what-you-eat-can-influence-how-you-sleep.

Anand P., A. B. Kunnumakkara, R. A. Newman, and B. B. Aggarwal. "Bioavailability of Curcumin: Problems and Promises." *Molecular Pharmacology*, no. 4. (2007): 807–18.

Bent, Stephen, et al. "Valerian for Sleep: A Systematic Review and Meta-Analysis." *American Journal of Medicine*, no. 119 (Dec. 2006): 1005–12.

Mao, Jun J., et al. "Long-Term Chamomile Therapy of Generalized Anxiety Disorder: A Study Protocol for a Randomized, Double-Blind, Placebo-Controlled Trial." *Journal of Clinical Trials*, no. 4 (Nov. 2014): 188.

St-Onge, Marie-Pierre, Amy Roberts, Ari Shechter, and Arindam Roy Choudhury. "Fiber and Saturated Fat Are Associated with Sleep Arousals and Slow Wave Sleep." *Journal of Clinical Sleep Medicine*, no. 12 (Jan. 2016): 19–24.

DIY

Mindell, Jodi, Lorena Telofski, Benjamin Wiegand, and Ellen Kurtz. "A Nightly Bedtime Routine: Impact on Sleep in Young Children and Maternal Mood." *Sleep*, no. 32 (May 2009): 599–606.

INDEX